MARY D. SHERIDAN'S PLAY IN EARLY CHILDHOOD

Mary D. Sheridan's Play in Early Childhood is a classic introductory text to play and development – key topics for all those who work with young children. Drawing on the most up-to-date evidence, it explains how children's play develops and how they develop as they play.

With over 100 illustrations and observations of play from birth to six years, this new edition presents classical and contemporary literature, making clear links between play and all areas of children's development. It includes updated activities to consolidate thinking and suggestions for further reading throughout. This text considers:

- the development, value and characteristics of play

- issues relating to culture, adversity, gender, attachment and brain development

- play from recreational, therapeutic and educational perspectives

- the role of parents/caregivers and professionals in supporting play

- how to develop observation and reflection skills for use in your own practice

Suitable both for those new to the area and for more experienced workers wanting a quick reference guide, this easy-to-follow book meets the needs of students and professionals from a wide range of health, education and social care backgrounds, including early years professionals, playworkers, children's nurses, play therapists and social workers.

Justine Howard is Associate Professor at the Centre for Child Research, Swansea University, UK, and a chartered psychologist. She is the programme director for the MA in Developmental and Therapeutic Play and the MA in Childhood Studies at Swansea and is also a consultant and trainer, providing continuing professional development in areas relating to child development, play and emotional health.

MARY D. SHERIDAN'S PLAY IN EARLY CHILDHOOD

From Birth to Six Years

Fourth Edition

Justine Howard

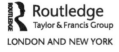

Routledge
Taylor & Francis Group

LONDON AND NEW YORK

First published 2017
by Routledge
2 Park Square, Milton Park, Abingdon, Oxon OX14 4RN

and by Routledge
711 Third Avenue, New York, NY 10017

Routledge is an imprint of the Taylor & Francis Group, an informa business

British Library Cataloguing-in-Publication Data
A catalogue record for this book is available from the British Library

Library of Congress Cataloging in Publication Data
A catalog record for this book has been requested.

ISBN: 978-1-138-65588-1 (hbk)
ISBN: 978-1-138-65591-1 (pbk)
ISBN: 978-1-315-62224-8 (ebk)

Typeset in Sabon
by Keystroke, Neville Lodge, Tettenhall, Wolverhampton

First photo on page 116 reproduced with kind permission of Lisa Morgan.

Contents

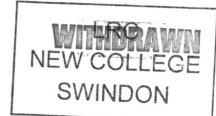

About the author

Justine Howard is a chartered psychologist and developmental and therapeutic play specialist. She has wide-ranging classroom experience and worked for a number of years alongside children with additional learning needs, before training in psychology and, later, in therapeutic play. She specializes in developmental psychology and the psychology of education. Her PhD focused on children's perceptions of their play and she has since spent more than 15 years researching this area. She is particularly interested in how play contributes to children's development and wellbeing. Her work has resulted in numerous publications, and she is widely considered an expert in the field. Justine is Associate Professor at Swansea University where she manages the MA in Developmental and Therapeutic Play and the MA in Childhood Studies.

Introduction

In his foreword to the original version of this book, Mary Sheridan's *Spontaneous Play in Early Childhood: From Birth to Six Years* (1977), Professor Jack Tizard described how at the time of Sheridan's writing, services concerned with children's intellectual, physical and social needs were grounded in knowledge about the nature of child development. Sheridan's observations of children's spontaneous play were invaluable in providing practitioners with an insight into the development of 'real children in real situations', allowing the reader to enrich their theoretical knowledge and validate their own experiences. This new edition continues to build on Sheridan's original work, maintaining her focus on the value of detailed observation for understanding key elements of children's development. It places her work in historical context whilst demonstrating its continued impact and currency in contemporary practice.

Play is recognized in Article 31 of the United Nations Convention on the Rights of the Child (United Nations, 1989), and the evidence base supporting the value of play for children's development, health and wellbeing continues to grow, contributing to a wide range of governmental policies. Not only do these policies relate directly to play, for example ensuring children have access to appropriate play experiences in health and social care, education and community spaces, but also to broader policies across children services relating to fitness, health, equal opportunities and reducing the poverty gap.

In 2015, a research centre dedicated to the study of children's play was opened at Cambridge University. Led by Dr. David Whitebread, the aim of the Centre for Research on Play in Education, Development and Learning (PEDAL) is to generate a substantial evidence base stemming from rigorous research that will inform theory, policy and practice in the UK and beyond. In the last five years, we have seen the launch of two new journals dedicated to the field of play, *The International Journal of Play* and *The Journal of Playwork Practice*. In addition, key articles relating to play and children's development have been published in highly regarded journals in related fields such as psychology and education, emphasizing the currency of play from an academic perspective and continued interest in the field.

Understanding children's development remains at the heart of services for children and knowledge about how and why play serves a critical developmental function is central to high-quality professional practice. Sheridan's focus was on spontaneity in play, characterized by the importance of freedom, choice and control. These features underpin the unique developmental potential of play and the practice of professionals working across contexts. In play, boundaries are set and regulated by children themselves. As a result, play promotes and protects esteem and maintains attention, optimizing opportunities for learning and development. *Learning through play* relies on children's *ability to play*, and understanding this, with reference to theories of child development and the detailed observations and illustrations (such as those of Sheridan), remains invaluable.

Sheridan was keen for her work not to be overly laden with controlled laboratory-type studies, which she believed detracted from the value of first hand naturalistic observations. I have tried to preserve this stance whilst at the same time, emphasizing the relationship between Sheridan's original observations, theories of play and development and current research evidence. This new edition aims to introduce readers to the fundamental relationship between play and aspects of children' development, allowing them to develop a personal philosophy of play that can guide their professional practice. There is added emphasis on the importance of key observation skills, difference and diversity in play and the importance of play for health and development across domains. The addition of photographs adds a contemporary feel to the text, which I hope enables readers to better relate Sheridan's seminal work to their own observations. Sheridan's work was motivated by her desire to ensure all children were provided with the highest level of care and support.

Readers will develop the knowledge and skills necessary to understand typical and atypical patterns in play and subsequently plan appropriate play experiences.

Professor Tizard acknowledged the special place of Mary Sheridan in British pediatrics, noting her as the most distinguished and senior practitioner in the field. She receives praise for the outstanding contribution of her work on the Royal Society of Medicine Wall of Honour. It goes without saying that everyone working across children's services should continue to benefit from her experience and expertise. Once again, it is a great privilege to have been asked to revise her work.

Justine Howard

1   Theorizing about play

Consistent with Sheridan's original work, this chapter will focus on definitions of play, functions of play and predominant play types. It will consider theories of play and evidence for the potential of play to support children's development across domains. In particular, it will highlight how the choice, control and ownership afforded to children during play enhances opportunities for learning and development.

The specific aims of the chapter are:

- To consider the issue of defining play and, in doing so, to highlight play as a *behaviour*, a *process* and an *approach to task*.

- To outline the importance of choice, control and ownership in children's play and to identify how the play cycle is maintained by signaling and responding to play cues.

- To consider why children play and what makes it valuable from a developmental perspective with reference to relevant theoretical accounts.

- To introduce the play types in which children typically engage and the sequence of play behaviour through which children typically progress.

- To highlight that play both influences and reflects children's development.

Defining play   When we begin to study any given concept or phenomenon, one of the first steps we take is to define what we understand that concept or phenomenon to mean. What is play and how is it different from other types of behaviour? While everyone has some idea about what it means to play and what play might look like, deciding on a clear and agreed definition has proven problematic. Indeed, it has been argued that play is so complex that it defies definition (Moyles, 1989; Lester & Russell, 2008; Howard & McInnes, 2013a). Considering the struggle to define play, however, provides an important narrative that reveals the complexity of play as a behaviour, a process and an approach to task. In particular, the freedom and choice inherent in spontaneous play make it a vital ingredient for children's healthy development.

Sheridan (1977) writes:

For the purpose of my own deliberations and discussions, I evolved the following:

- *Play* is the eager engagement in pleasurable physical or mental effort to obtain emotional satisfaction.

- *Work* is the voluntary engagement in disciplined physical or mental effort to obtain material benefit.

- *Drudgery* is the enforced engagement in distasteful physical or mental effort to obtain the means of survival.

- We all know that play and work may merge into each other (I would define this as *ploy*), and work and drudgery may also merge (I would define this as *slog*), but play and drudgery are incompatible.

- The everyday world of school children provides a foretaste of the adult world in that their daily work consists of uneven and fluctuating combinations of ploy, acquired competence and slog, just as our own work consists of varying amounts of exciting research, skilled practices and pedestrian plodding.

Dictionary definitions of play suggest it is characterized by being frivolous, fun or light-hearted. However, this is at odds with the deep seriousness that can often be apparent when we observe children at play (Lester & Russell, 2008). Some theorists have suggested

Play as a behaviour

that for an activity to be regarded as play, certain characteristics must be observed. For example, Krasnor and Pepler (1980) suggest that for an activity to be defined as play, we must observe voluntary participation, enjoyment, intrinsic motivation, pretence and a focus on process over product. A problem with this type of approach, however, is that while these characteristics might be clearly evident in some instances of play, in other situations they are more difficult, if not impossible, to identify. Pellegrini (1991) proposes that the more characteristics that are present, the more 'like play' the activity becomes. However, what if some of these characteristics are more important to an activity being play-like than others? What if two different observers see things differently? For example, one observer might believe that an activity being voluntary is far more important than it not having an end product, whereas another observer might make their decision based on signs of fun and enjoyment. Let's consider two examples of children playing with Lego blocks.

- Child (A) takes the blocks from the toy shelf in their bedroom. They take them to the table and become intently focused on building a replica of the model presented on the box packaging. There is no laughter or smiling; they appear lost in concentration, searching for the pieces and frequently glancing towards the box, checking if their structure is the same as the one pictured.

- Child (B) is handed the Lego blocks by their teacher and they take them to the carpet. They appear to be haphazardly building the bricks, the structure takes no particular form, and they change what they do as they go along. Sometimes they organize the bricks into piles by colour. Sometimes they put the bricks in piles according to size. They occasionally smile and laugh as they build up the bricks and then knock them down.

Which of these activities would be defined as play? Child (A) chose to take part in the activity, there is clearly an end product and there are no overt signs of pleasure and enjoyment. The activity was chosen for Child (B), they showed signs that the activity was enjoyable and fun and they didn't appear to be working towards any end product or goal. Neither of the scenarios demonstrates any element of pretence.

In fact, both of the children in the scenarios above described their activities as play. This highlights how seeing play from an adult perspective or making a decision as to what is and what isn't play based on observation can be problematic. All too often, our approach to defining play is based on adult views of what play looks like, rather than taking the child's perspective (Holt *et al.*, 2015). Play means different things to different people at different times (Howard, 2009; Howard & McInnes, 2013a). For example, the 'play' of the professional footballer will be very different from the 'play' that occurs between friends at an after-school knock-around (Saracho, 1990). To understand play, we need to find out what players themselves think about the nature of their activities. Various types of play activity are detailed later in this chapter, but it is not enough for activities to look like play. We also need to understand what makes children approach activities in a playful way. Evidence suggests that much of the developmental potential of play relies on children approaching an activity in a playful way (e.g. Miller & Kuhaneck, 2008; McInnes *et al.*, 2009; McInnes *et al.*, 2013; Howard & McInnes, 2013b).

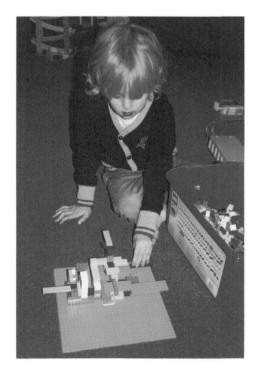

This young boy is busy building a Lego model, but can we be certain that he thinks the activity is play?

Play as an approach to task

Until quite recently, little research had focused on children's own perceptions of their play. Studies that have investigated what play means to children, however, have been fruitful and have led to much deeper insight as to what separates play from other types of activity. Such studies have featured in international reports relating to the importance of play (e.g. Lester & Russell, 2008; Whitebread, 2012), have influenced play policy (e.g. CSFC, 2010) and have informed the planning and provision for play across children's services (e.g. Millar & Kuhaneck, 2008; Brockman *et al.*, 2011; Holt *et al.*, 2015).

Research demonstrates that preschool children define play as activity that is freely chosen and self-directed. Surprisingly, young children do not often define play as being something that is necessarily fun (Robson, 1993; Keating *et al.*, 2000). This differs from the views of children in middle childhood, where at aged seven to nine years, fun becomes a more important feature (King & Howard, 2014; Brockman *et al.*, 2011; Howard *et al.*, 2017).

In addition to choice and control, for children in the early years, activities that occur on the floor, rather than at a table, and outside, rather than inside, are more likely to be seen as play (Howard, 2002; Parker, 2007). The nature and degree of adult involvement in young children's play is also important (McInnes *et al.*, 2011). Bundy (1993) argues that the way children approach an activity may be far more important than the actual activity itself. The same activity might be described by children as play or not play, depending on the freedom, choice and control they are afforded.

Play and exploration

The characteristics associated with play and non-play become particularly important when children enter a nursery or classroom situation and they begin to experience structured activities. It is here where we begin to see them comparing play with work activity in the way suggested by Sheridan. However, what about the play of babies and infants who have yet to make a distinction between play and other types of activity? Piaget (1951) and Hutt (1976) propose that activity progresses from exploration to play as children become familiar with objects and their environments. At the exploration stage, children are finding out what an object does, whereas during play, they begin to consider what they can do with

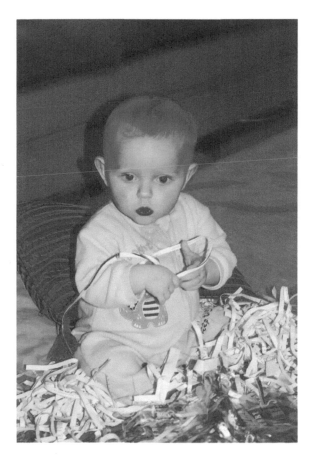

Sensory experiences are an important precursor to play. This baby is deeply engaged, exploring the texture, colour and sound of shredded paper.

that object. Much of the activity we can observe in young infants might be categorized as exploration (Pellegrini & Gustafson, 2005). This exploration is comparable from a developmental perspective to the more structured learning experienced in later childhood. Early exploration is important, as it acts as a springboard for the development of future play skills. In her EPR model of play development, Jennings (1999) defines this initial sensory exploration of objects and the environment as 'Embodied play' (E) and proposes that it is the first stage in the development of play skills, where children learn to distinguish a sense of self as separate to others. Knowing that the self is separate to other people and things is a necessary step toward allowing one object to stand for *something else* in symbolic projective play (P) and finally *someone else* in role play (R).

This little one has no understanding about the function of the abacus but is exploring how it moves, sounds and feels.

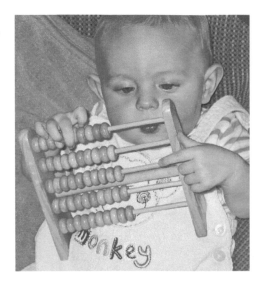

The dynamic process of play

Play is a behaviour, an approach to task, but also a process. Children move in and out of play according to their own needs and wishes and other influences within the environment. Other influences on children's play might include location, the availability of materials, time and the involvement of other people (King & Howard, 2014). Sturrock and Else (1998) suggest that play is a cycle of activity (as can be seen in Figure 1). They propose that children communicate the desire to play using a series of signals and that for play to maintain momentum these signals must be responded to appropriately.

Perhaps the simplest example of this is one child inviting another to engage in a game of catch. Throwing a ball to another child might be seen as a signal or invitation to engage in the game. The second child receives and responds to the signal and the ball is thrown back and forth. Then, one child decides they no longer wish to play the game, and they stop returning the ball. The signal to play isn't responded to, and the play comes to an end. Alternatively, the second child may decide they want to change the nature of the game, and so they begin to bounce rather than throw the ball. They invite the original child to engage in a new game. If the original child bounces the ball back, they accept the game change and the cycle continues. If not, they might either revert back to their original throwing behaviour in a bid to maintain the flow or end the play completely.

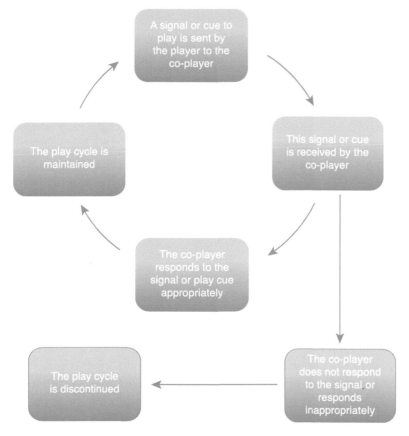

Figure 1 The play cycle

A signal or cue to play is sent by the player to the co-player

This signal or cue is received by the co-player

The play cycle is maintained

The co-player responds to the signal or play cue appropriately

The play cycle is discontinued

The co-player does not respond to the signal or responds inappropriately

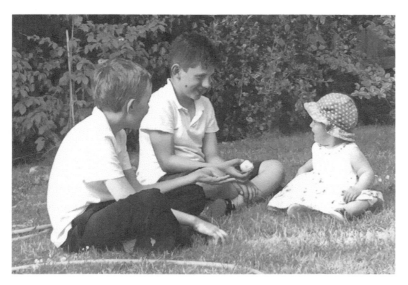

At an early age, children start to understand play signals. These two young boys were very pleased when the baby finally started to throw the ball back and forth.

In order to maintain a state of play, the needs and wishes of the players are negotiated. This process is similar to the flow state identified by Csikszentmihalyi and Csikszentmihalyi (1988), where a sense of choice and control over the activity leads to deep concentration, pleasure and satisfaction.

Functions of play

Sheridan's focus was on children's *spontaneous* play, suggesting a natural inclination or drive towards play activity. This intrinsic motivation is reflected in reviews documenting the importance of play for children's learning and development (Lester & Russell, 2010; Whitebread, 2012; APPG, 2015). Early philosophical accounts explain the spontaneous drive towards play as being the result of evolution or biological functioning:

- *Pre-exercise theory* (Groos, 1901) suggests that play behaviour exists as a means of practising key skills that are essential to adult survival.

- *Recapitulation theory* (Hall, 1920) suggests that in play, children act out behaviours that were once essential for human survival but are no longer necessary, such as building dens or climbing trees.

- *Relaxation theory* (Patrick, 1916) suggests that we are driven to play because it involves minimal cognitive demands. Periods of play allow us to relax, storing energy in preparation for more important cognitive activity.

- *Surplus energy theory* (Spencer, 1898) suggests that play allows us to release excess energy that has not been spent fulfilling survival needs. As children are largely looked after by others, their unspent energy levels are high, resulting in the propensity to play.

Providing evidence as to why children seem to have a natural inclination towards play is difficult. It seems likely that there is a combination of reasons as to why play is children's preferred mode of action. Children certainly seem motivated to explore the world around them and to make sense of their experiences, and the development of their play skills seems to stem from this motivation. From their earliest sensory experiences and interactions with others, children develop a repertoire of play skills that support their development. Of importance is that children choose to learn about the world through play, and a sense of choice remains an important element of their play throughout childhood. Evidence from research in middle childhood, however, indicates that contrary to widely held beliefs, activities do not have to be entirely freely chosen, and children accept activities as play even where they have made compromises as to where, when and with whom they play (King & Howard, 2014).

There is widespread recognition that children's play serves a useful developmental function. Whilst based largely on animal studies, the field of neuroscience has begun to explore the notion that enriched or playful experiences support the development of the growing brain (see Lester & Russell, 2008; Whitebread, 2012). Jarvis, Newman and Swiniarski (2014) suggest that play helps to promote the development of neuronal structures that, in particular, contribute to emotional health and sociability. In their neurosequential model of therapeutic intervention, Perry, Hogan and Marlin (2000) propose that the development of children's play behaviour mirrors the development of specific regions of the brain. The role of play in promoting and supporting development has become a principal focus for scholars in multiple disciplines and for a wide variety of professionals across children's services. We have seen the introduction of policies dedicated to ensuring that children have appropriate opportunities to play from an educational, recreational and health care perspective, and the importance of play is recognized in Article 31 of the United Nations Convention on the Rights of the Child (United Nations, 1989). The specific role of play for learning, recreation, health and wellbeing is discussed further in chapter 5.

Sheridan's recognition of the value of play in relation to the whole child is echoed in recent documentation such as *Best Play* (Department for Culture, Media and Sport, 2000), which states that during play children learn and develop as individuals but also as members of the wider community. It also features widely across policies relating to children's health and wellbeing (APPG, 2015).

Sheridan (1977) writes:

A child's developmental progress may be conveniently observed and defined within the context of the following parameters:

- *Motor development* involving body postures and large movements. These combine high physical competence and economy of effort with precise forward planning in time and space.

- *Vision and fine movements* involving competence in seeing and looking (far and near) and manipulative skills, integrating sensory, motor, tactile and proprioceptive activities.

- *Hearing and listening* and the *use of codes of communication.*

- *Social behaviour and spontaneous play* involving competence in organization of the self (i.e. self-identity, self-care and self-occupation), together with voluntary acceptance of cultural standards regarding personal behaviour and social demands.

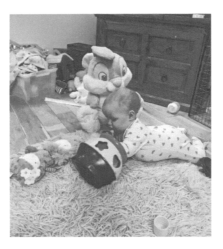 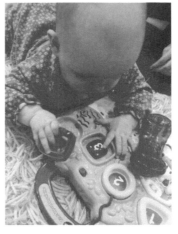

At 6 months, now strong enough to hold herself up on her arms for a considerable time, this little one was deeply engaged putting the blocks in and out of their container.

At 8 months, she learned that she could make lights and sounds by pressing the numbered buttons on her new toy.

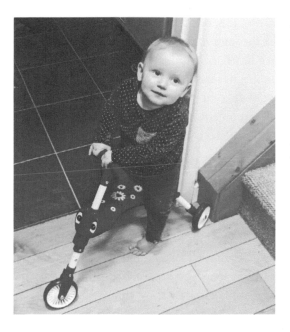

At 15 months, after having mastered balancing herself on the small trike, she began to learn how to move, for a long time only propelling herself backwards. At 18 months, steering remained a challenge.

■ *Social and emotional development.* In play, children have the opportunity to learn about themselves and others. They become aware of the impact of their behaviour and develop skills in conflict resolution, negotiation, trust and acceptance. They can *try out* different ways of dealing with social situations and *try on* feelings, emotions and social roles.

■ *Cognitive development.* Play offers opportunities to learn about objects, concepts and ideas: for example, sorting, sequencing, weight and balance. Children develop problem-solving strategies, and the ability to allow one thing to stand for something else (for example, in pretend play) is a precursor to more complex ways of thinking.

■ *Language development.* Play offers opportunities for the development of language skill in relation to vocabulary, pronunciation, sentence construction and the transmission of meaning and intent.

■ *Physical development.* Play involves gross and fine motor movements and as such promotes co-ordination and visuo-spatial ability. The increased aerobic activity resulting from sustained active play promotes physical health and fitness in terms of the cardiovascular system, muscle tone and maintenance of optimum weight.

However, children learn in lots of different ways: for example, via imitation, by rote and through direct instruction. A key question for those studying play has been to identify what makes learning through play so valuable. Researchers have sought to be able to show that play, rather than other types of activity, makes a difference to children's development. With this in mind, we begin to appreciate the importance of clearly defining what play actually is.

Significant advances in evidencing the benefits of play have been made by focusing on children's own perceptions of their play. It has allowed researchers to compare children's behaviour and performance during the same task where conditions are manipulated to be more or less like play (according to children's own views). This powerful research has shown that when children perceive an activity as play rather than not play, their performance in problem-solving tasks is significantly improved, and they show much deeper levels of engagement and motivation (McInnes *et al.*, 2009; McInnes *et al.*, 2011). Ring (2010) found that encouraging a playful approach to drawing in the early years by offering children freedom, choice and control led to increased participation and progress in their ability to use drawing as a tool for meaning making and communication. During activities that are play, children show higher levels of meta-cognition and self-regulation, a finding replicated in later work (Whitebread, 2010; Bryce & Whitebread, 2012). In addition, Howard & McInnes (2013b) demonstrated that despite the type of activity remaining constant (e.g. completing a jigsaw puzzle), when children felt the activity was play (e.g. where they were offered choice, allowed to do the activity where they wished and without adult direction), they showed increased signs of emotional wellbeing.

These findings are consistent with the proposition that taking a playful approach to a task is far more important than the task itself (Bundy, 1993). While children learn in a number of different ways, their learning is enhanced across all developmental domains when an activity is approached as play. Sutton-Smith (1974) and Bruner (1979) suggest that playful activity is particularly beneficial for children's development, as it promotes flexible thinking skills, an idea that has been extended in playwork practice through the compound flexibility theory of Brown (2003). Howard and Miles (2008) suggest that the differences in behaviour and improved performance exhibited when children approach tasks as play is a result of reduced behavioural thresholds. When children are in a playful mode, outcomes are flexible and fear is reduced, and consequently, more potential behaviours become available to try out. A sense of freedom, choice and control in play means that boundaries are set and regulated by children themselves. As a result, play promotes and protects esteem and maintains attention for learning to take place (Howard, 2010a).

Types of play

It is important to note that play both influences and reflects development. Some typologies of play document the activities we are likely to see children engaging in throughout the course of their childhoods. We can note how these different types of play are contributing to development. These typologies can be simplistic or complex.

Hutt (1976) proposes a distinction between *epistemic* play, which focuses on the acquisition of knowledge and skill, and *ludic* play, which is more concerned with fantasy and make believe.

In contrast, Hughes (1999) has compiled an extensive typology that describes 16 different play types:

- *Rough and tumble* — encounter activity involving touch, tickling and the use of relative strength with an indication that the activity is play

- *Socio-dramatic* — the enactment of real and potential human experience

- *Social* — play with rules for social engagement

- *Creative* — play that facilitates a number of potential outcomes or responses

- *Communication* — play using words, nuances or gestures

- *Dramatic* — play that dramatizes events in which the child is not a direct participant

- *Symbolic* — play where one thing can stand for another

- *Deep* — play that allows the child to encounter risky experiences

- *Exploratory* — play to access factual information about objects or concepts

- *Fantasy* — play that rearranges the world in the child's way, a way that is unlikely to occur

- *Imaginative* — play where the conventional rules that govern the physical world do not apply

- *Locomotor* — movement in any or every direction for its own sake

- *Mastery* — control of the physical and affective ingredients of the environment

- *Object* — play that uses infinite and interesting sequences of hand–eye manipulations and movements

- *Role* — play exploring ways of being, although not normally of an intense personal, social, domestic or interpersonal nature

- *Recapitulative* — play that allows the child to explore ancestry, history, rituals, stories, rhymes, fire and darkness

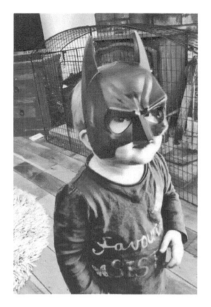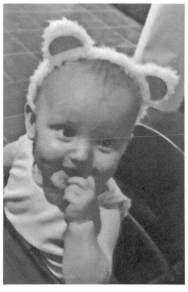

From an early age, children enjoy dressing up. As they get older, role play becomes increasingly complex to include detailed scripts and narratives.

This little one gets a reaction from others when she puts on the mask and ears and so repeats the action multiple times. However, she doesn't really understand how it changes her appearance.

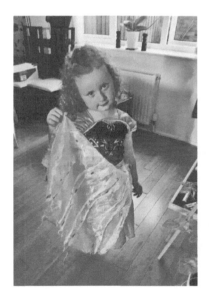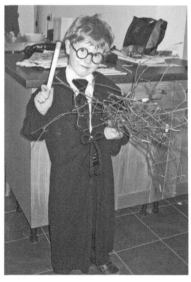

At around three years old, this little girl recognises that putting on this costume turns her into a princess.

At six years, dress up play can lead to the acting out of roles with stories and narratives.

Other typologies of play have a more developmental focus and outline progression through certain play types as children acquire a growing repertoire of skills. Here the focus is on how children develop their ability to play. Whitebread (2012) suggests that across cultures, there are five main play types: physical play, play with objects, symbolic play, pretence/sociodramatic play and games with rules. These resonate with the original observations of Sheridan that are highlighted below.

Sheridan (1977) writes:

Different types of play emerge in developmental sequence as the child learns to use first their sensory and motor equipment to best advantage and later their powers of communication and creativity. Every step forward depends upon successful achievement of previous stepping-stones.

1 **Active play** presumes 'gross motor' control of head, trunk and limbs in sitting, crawling, standing, running, climbing, jumping, throwing, kicking, catching and so on. It is directly concerned with promotion of physical development and necessitates the provision of adequate free-ranging space to move about in and natural obstacles to overcome, together with simple, safe, playground equipment, mobile and fixed.

2 **Exploratory and manipulative play**, beginning at about 3 months with finger-play, presumes possession of age-appropriate gross-motor, fine-motor and sensory functioning. These components are essential not only for acquisition of hand–eye co-ordination but also for attending to and localizing everyday sounds, for recognition of the permanence of objects and for learning to appreciate the implications of space and time. Integration of these separate physical and cognitive elements into total meaningful experience necessitates the availability of a number of simple things for manipulation,

such as everyday domestic objects as well as traditional playthings like rattles, dolls, balls, building blocks, boxes, toys to grasp and move about by hand and sound-making instruments.

3 **Imitative play** becomes clearly evident from 7–9 months. It presumes a child's ability to control their body, manipulate objects, integrate and interpret multisensorial experience and comprehend simple language, or perhaps more accurately, their caregivers' vocal tunes. It reflects what a child sees and hears going on around them, providing a lively record of their perceptual learning. At first, this imitation is fragmentary and follows immediately upon the child's attention being attracted in some way to the activity that they imitate. Later, they recall and repeat for their own amusement or for applause a series of these meaningful actions. Imitative play is necessary in order for a child not only to learn the quickest and most effective way of performing meaningful actions themselves but also gradually to understand that adults have differing roles and responsibilities.

4 **Constructive (or end-product) play,** beginning with very simple block-building at about 18–20 months, presumes possession of all the aforementioned motor and sensory abilities together with increasing capacity to make use of the intellectual processes involved in recognition and retrieval of previously stored memories. Additionally, it requires ability to create preliminary 'blueprints' in the mind and realize these in practical form. This type of play grows directly out of early exploratory and manipulative play but also implies capacity to combine early 'pure' imitation with purposeful anticipation.

5 **Make-believe (or pretend) play,** beginning a couple of months before 2 years and elaborated for several years afterwards, presumes previous acquisition of all the foregoing

types, particularly imitative role play. Having learned from experience the probable causes and effects relating to the activities they have observed and copied, children now deliberately invent increasingly complex make-believe situations for themselves in order to practise and enjoy their acquired insights and skills. In this way, they improve their general knowledge and, most importantly of all, refine their social communications. Make-believe play depends upon a child's ability to receive and express their ideas in some form of language-code. Consequently, its spontaneous employment is of considerable diagnostic significance to professional workers concerned with the health, welfare and education of young children.

6 **Games-with-rules** presuppose a high degree of skill in all the foregoing types, including full understanding and acceptance of the abstractions involved in sharing, taking turns, fair play and accurate recording of results. They usually start at about four years when small groups of peerage children, under tacitly acknowledged leadership, improvise their own rules for co-operative play. Team games, which challenge competitiveness in older children and adults, become increasingly subject to rules imposed from without and, to be rewarding, must be played strictly according to the recognized constitution.

Sheridan observes how children's spontaneous play changes over time, and the types of play she describes are consistent with theorists who suggest that play follows a developmental trajectory. It is generally accepted that the ages associated with any stage theory of development are approximate; however, as described earlier in this chapter with reference to embodied, projective and role play (Jennings, 1999), of importance is the sequence in which behaviours emerge. The behaviours predominantly associated with one stage may occur concurrently with another, and the play behaviours are cumulative rather than exclusive. The progressive nature

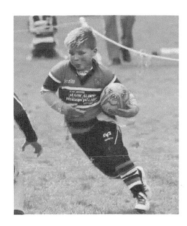

As well as promoting physical health, rugby provides opportunities for children to learn about rules, co-operation and being part of a team.

of play has been documented from a cognitive, social and emotional perspective.

Piaget (1951) proposed three stages of play that corresponded with cognitive development:

- *Practice play*: In the sensorimotor stage of development (approximately birth to two years), children explore their own bodies and the objects around them using sight, sound, touch and taste; the play here is often repetitive.

- *Symbolic play*: Early in the pre-operational stage (approximately two to seven years), children develop the ability to allow one thing to stand for another, and pretend play or make believe begins to emerge.

- *Games with rules*: In the latter part of the pre-operational stage of development and into the concrete operational stage (approximately aged seven to eleven years), play becomes increasingly governed by rules.

Throughout childhood, play provides opportunities for children to learn about their physical abilities. Older children become increasingly competitive, this six-year-old was very pleased to be able to hula-hoop for longer than his older sister!

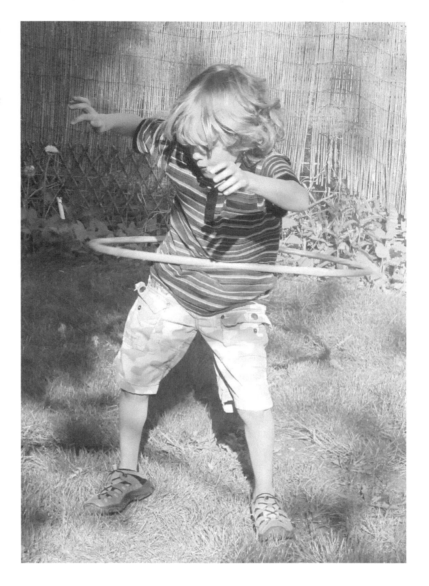

Parten (1932) observed children aged two to five years in their pre-school environment. Through extensive observations, she noted that play became increasingly social with age. She described six social stages of play:

■ *Unoccupied behaviour*: Not playing, simply observing

■ *Solitary play*: Child plays alone, uninterested in others

- *Onlooker behaviour*: Child watches the play of others and may talk to the children involved but this talk does not relate to the play

- *Parallel play*: Child plays alongside others, often imitating what is being played nearby, but no interaction

- *Associative play*: The children appear to be playing together but their activities are not organized

- *Co-operative play*: Playing together in more organized activities where they share intentions about the progress of the play

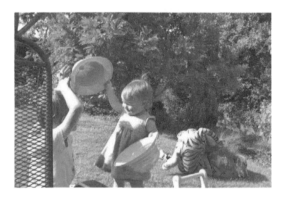

These two youngsters spent a short time engaged in associative play being jungle explorers. It was not long, however, before they became distracted. In parallel, one played with his baby sister whilst the other wrestled with the tiger.

Erikson (1963) focused on the emotional benefits of play and suggested that children's play served as a means of developing a sense of competence and positive self-esteem:

- *Autocosmic play*: During the first year of life, of most significance to Erikson was that early play focused on the child's exploration of the body and the senses. Awareness of the bodily self was seen as an important precursor to self-esteem in that we cannot evaluate the self without first having a basic awareness of what that self comprises.

- *Microspheric play*: In their second year, children begin to play with objects, and during this time, they begin to understand the impact that their own actions can have on the environment.

■ *Macrospheric play*: At around three years, when children may enter preschool or nursery, play becomes more social. Activities are shared, and children become aware that their environment and their sense of self are not only controlled by themselves but are influenced by others. They learn how to maintain a positive sense of self in the wider social world.

At 6 months, this little one is not yet aware that the reflection she can see in the mirror is herself. She reaches out to touch the 'other baby' in just the same way as she does with her baby massage friend.

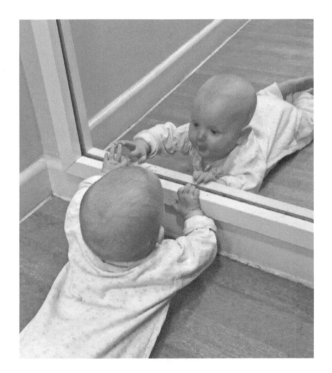

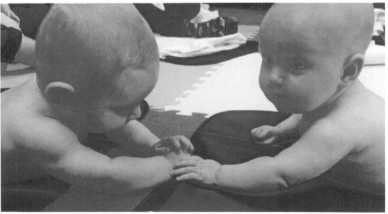

Summary

■ Play reflects but also supports children's development.

■ Play is more than just a behaviour; it is a process and a way of approaching an activity.

■ Children are more likely to approach an activity as play when they are afforded freedom, choice and control.

■ Development is enhanced when children approach activities as play.

Observe a child or group of children engaged in play.

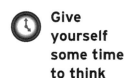

Give yourself some time to think

■ Why do you think the activity is play?

■ Do you think the children would agree? Why?

  – Can you see evidence of the play cycle?

■ In what ways do you think this play reflects and supports children's development?

Useful reading

Brown, S. (2009) *Play: How it shapes the brain, opens the imagination and invigorates the soul.* New York: Avery.

Howard, J. & McInnes, K. (2013a) *The essence of play: A practice companion for professionals working with children and young people.* London: Routledge.

Whitebread, D. (2012) *The importance of play: A report on the value of children's play with policy recommendations.* Brussels: Toys Industry Europe.

2 Observing and reflecting on children at play

This chapter considers the importance of developing key observational skills in order to be able to reflect accurately on children's behaviour. It presents a historical overview of the study of children's development, demonstrating an increasingly systematic and scientific approach. The chapter focus is mainly confined to the consideration of small-scale naturalistic observational methods, as this is the approach that was predominantly used by Sheridan to inform her work. The benefits of systematic observation are highlighted and some simple examples of how this can be achieved are outlined. These examples of observational methods are presented with reference to some of the observations made by Sheridan throughout this book.

The specific aims of the chapter are:

■ To discuss the history of studying children's development and the emergence of childhood as a specific area of scientific interest

■ To highlight some of the reasons why developing observation skills is important in informing theory, policy and practice relating to children

■ To consider some examples of observational methods that can help us to reflect accurately on children's behaviour

The history of observing children and childhood

Childhood has not always been regarded as a stage of development that is unique, distinct and worthy of study. By considering changes in how childhood has been conceptualized through different periods in time, we can note a move from what could be described as a time where children were regarded as merely miniature, to a time where the complexity of their development has been increasingly regarded as miraculous. In the preformationist period that was dominant up until the 18th century, children were regarded as miniature versions of adults, growing only in a physical sense. They were thought to be 'preformed', even from the point of conception where it was believed that the sperm implanted into the womb was itself, a fully formed human but in miniature form. There are some wonderful illustrations of this concept in sketches created by Leonardo da Vinci that are well worth seeking out. From this perspective, it is easy to understand why children were treated as they were, dressed in adult clothing and not given any special attention. There was no particular provision for play and children were often tasked with adult responsibilities from an early age. With the development of equipment that enabled scientific study, initially and simplistically the microscope, such ideas were gradually dispelled, and more complex theories of development began to emerge.

The Age of Enlightenment contributed to changes in our conceptualisation of childhood and influential thinkers such as Locke (1632–1704) and Rousseau (1712–1778) described their philosophical ideas about human development. Locke believed that children were born as 'tabula rasa' or 'blank slates', upon which perceptual experiences became imprinted. Environmental experiences shaped the mind through association, repetitive exposure, imitation, reward and punishment. Rousseau focused more on the social determinants of development, arguing that the child was a 'noble savage' with a propensity to act on impulse. These initial impulses were gradually brought into line by social forces and the need for compliance. He saw development as occurring in stages, beginning with sensory learning in infancy, the growth of independence and emergent reasoning in early childhood, significant physical and cognitive change in later childhood with the mature social beings emerging in adolescence. Whilst these were philosophical accounts and not based on supporting evidence, we can clearly see how these ideas relate to central theories of development that emerged throughout the nineteenth and twentieth centuries. The Age of Enlightenment was marked by other advances in science, industry and society and from this, there stemmed a growing academic interest in exploring children's development.

Some of the earliest accounts of children's development were the result of baby biographers, perhaps the most famous of these being Charles Darwin. Darwin (1809–1882) wrote a detailed diary of his children's behaviours from birth to three years and used these observations to support his evolutionary theory of development, describing, for example, how thinking skills grew from those that were simple to those that were complex over time. The publication of this work led to considerable growth in research focused on children's development across domains (Lorch & Hellal, 2010). The limitations of single case study observations however, were soon much discussed. Scientists began to question issues such as subjectivity and bias, the difficulties associated with replicating findings and whether findings could realistically be generalized to the wider population. As a result there was rapid growth in new approaches to data collection. This included collecting data from large samples, developing standardized tests or controlled experimental procedures, often favouring laboratory studies over those conducted in naturalistic settings.

Piaget (1896–1980) combined naturalistic observations with experimental procedures to develop his influential theory of child development. His ideas on the development and function of play are detailed in chapter 1. Observations of his own children provided the basis for his theoretical ideas and were of great significance. Below is one of his diary entries about his daughter, demonstrating an example of imitation.

> At 0:4(23) without any previous practice I showed L my hand which I was slowly opening and closing. She seemed to be imitating me. All the time my suggestion lasted she kept up a similar movement to me and either stopped or did something else as soon as I stopped. (Piaget, 1951, 23)

Further extracts from his diary entries demonstrate the lengths he went to, to systematically identify the reasons behind his daughter's behaviour, experimenting with new ideas and explanations.

> There was the same reaction when I repeated the action at 0:4(26) but was this response of L merely trying an attempt

at prehension [the act of trying to grasp something]. To test this, I then showed her some other object. She again opened and closed her hand but only twice, then immediately tried to seize the object and suck it. I resumed the action with my hand and she clearly imitated it, her gesture being quite different from the one she had made on seeing the toy. (Ibid.)

Mary Sheridan (1899–1978) acknowledged the value of standardized tests and controlled experiments but also recognized the limitations of these methods that arguably, at the time, were in a relatively embryonic state. Her experiences of working with children from diverse populations, and with differing health and development concerns, led her to question whether such measures alone could universally describe children's development and specifically identify at the earliest opportunity when additional care and support may be required.

[Sheridan] soon saw that . . . it was essential to be thoroughly familiar with developmental progress in infancy and early childhood and more particularly with the range of normality. From practical experience she found that the accepted tests of children's intelligence and maturation were in many ways inadequate. This drove her to discover for herself what the normal parameters of a child's development should be at different ages and how best to detect handicapping conditions in their earliest stages. (Hamilton, 2016, para 2.)

Sheridan set about undertaking an extensive series of systematic observations, from which she developed her own developmental screening methods (STYCAR). The STYCAR sequences (Sheridan, 1978) were subsequently used to inform the Schedule of Growing Skills or SOGS, as they have become known (Belmann, Lungain & Ankett, 1996). Testament to Sheridan's acute observational skills, these remain active in professional practice to the current day.

The importance of observations for informing theory, policy and practice

Understanding children's development is important. Observations feed into an evidence-based cycle that informs theory, policy and professional practice (Figure 2). To provide the best quality health, care and developmental support for children, we need to have detailed knowledge of children's developmental progress in relation to social and emotional, language, physical and cognitive skills. Whilst this need not be exact in relation to age of acquisition, nor focus unnecessarily on what children are able or unable to achieve, such knowledge is important as it allows us to best plan for children's individual needs, providing optimum environmental opportunities.

Play is a particularly useful domain for observing and assessing children's development, as arguably it is their natural occupation. As such, it is a place where children not only feel safe to be themselves but also, are more likely as a result of this self-directed environment, to exhibit skills that best reflect (or even exceed) their abilities. This is in contrast to formal testing situations, where children may be likely to under achieve as a result of feeling threatened by the fear of failure (Epstein *et al.*, 2004). Observing children at play helps us

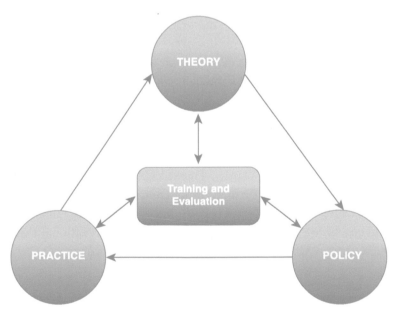

Figure 2 The cycle of evidence-based practice

to understand how play behaviour evolves over time and also provides an opportunity to consider children's developmental progress across domains. Detailed knowledge of children's progress in play has facilitated the development of formal play based assessments that can be used to support practitioners in providing appropriate play opportunities. Some examples include the Penn Interactive Peer Play Scale (PIPPS) that considers social interaction skills during play, the Developmental Play Assessment (DPA) that tracks children's behaviour to give an overview of their current play level and the Play Observation Scale (POS) based on the work of Piaget and Parten's theories of social and cognitive development.

Observing children at play enabled Sheridan to document patterns of developmental progress in play, but also, demonstrate how play reflected key advances in social, physical and cognitive skills. She gathered her information through authentic and naturalistic observations of play where children are likely to be in their most engaged and motivated state (Howard & McInnes, 2013).

There are a variety of ways that we can study children's development. This could include case studies where a single child is observed over a designated period of time, studies that involve groups of children in a particular age range, or longitudinal cohort studies that document development over several years. An example of the latter is the Millennium Cohort Study funded by the Economic Social Research Council that is tracking the development of 19,000 children from the United Kingdom born in the year 2000, from birth through to adulthood (see the Centre for Longitudinal Studies at www.cls.ioe.ac.uk).

Undertaking child observations

We can gather information about children's development in numerous ways, for example using diaries, self-developed observation schedules, charts which note the frequency of certain behaviours or standardized measures or tests such as those detailed earlier in the section above. There are strengths and limitations to the approaches we choose that can influence how informative the findings of our observations are. For example, whether we can be sure the behaviours we have observed are typical or whether other factors might account for what has been observed. These issues will determine whether we can generalize our findings to a wider population.

When undertaking observations, regardless of how structured or controlled our approach to gathering data, or whether our observation involves a single child or group of children, there are key considerations that can ensure we make the most of our time and efforts.

Being prepared and systematic

The first steps in undertaking an observation are important ones. They will help to ensure that appropriate information is collected. Consider what the purpose of the observation is and choose a method of observation that allows this purpose to be met. For example, if the purpose of the observation is to assess a child's developmental progress, then a standardized measure may be a suitable approach. If the aim is to evaluate the success of a particular area of the playroom or a play activity, then you might choose to develop your own observation schedule that notes how often children use the area, how long they play there and what they do. If you are interested in observing age related characteristics of children's play, you may chose to document how they behave in a variety of different play situations in relation to one or many areas of development. You will need to decide whether observing one or multiple children best suits the needs of your aim. If you decide to observe a group of children, then you will need to decide when each child will be observed and how you will ensure that each child is observed for the same length of time in a similar range of contexts.

Being accurate and objective

Once the aim of the observation is determined and an approach to gathering data has been chosen, it is important to be mindful of accuracy and objectivity. Our observations should note exactly what is seen, with any personal inferences of what this might mean being clearly marked as being separate to the actual observation itself. It is important to be aware of how prior knowledge and expectations can influence or *bias* what we believe we are seeing. If we are involved with the children during the observation process then it is important to understand how our interactions can be influential in shaping how children behave. As much relevant detail as possible should be provided, it is better to have too much information than too little. Some types of observation will allow the completion of checklists or short notes in situ, other approaches might require notes to be written after the event. There are strengths and limitations of immediate and retrospective documentation. If we take notes during an observation, this could interrupt the observation itself. If notes are written retrospectively, they could be more prone to error, subjectivity and inference.

There are basic details that need to be recorded on all observations, for example details about the child (age, gender, any relevant family or cultural details along with any relevant health or developmental details). For confidentiality purposes, it is good practice to anonymise these details (using an identifier or pseudonym) and to ensure that information is kept in a secure location. Parents or guardians should be fully informed about the observation and give consent for their child to take part. In addition, we need to note when and where the observation was conducted. Other details that could also influence a child's behaviour might also be useful. Whether the child is familiar with the environment (and the observer) could be important as, might be the time of day (for example, behaviour might be impacted by tiredness or hunger). Changes to routine should also be documented, for example if there is a new teacher or adult in the environment. Sheridan supported her observations by taking photographs of children's activities that were subsequently turned into line drawings for publication. Photographs of what children create can be a source of useful supporting evidence for observations. If photographs of children are taken, it is important that we gain explicit permission for this, describing to parents their purpose, the way they will be used and how / whether they will be shared with others.

Noting all relevant and supporting details

Sheridan used her observations to identify sequences of play with particular objects, developmental progress in play and the skills and abilities children exhibit during their play activities. In this section we will reflect on Sheridan's observations and consider some of the approaches she might have taken to gather her data and make inferences about children's play behaviours.

Some simple systematic approaches to observing children's play

Observations of children at play will most often be naturalistic (occurring in the child's normal daily environment) rather than being laboratory based. It is possible however, to offer particular

Diary entries and running records

experiences or materials for play, so that specific behaviours can be observed. Sheridan observed how children engaged with particular objects at different ages. She incorporated her observations into descriptions of play sequences that involved a cup, bell and blocks, small world toys and mark making. These sequences are described in chapter 4.

Narrative approaches such as diary entries or running records are very suited to observing how children interact with particular objects over time. A diary method involves observing children's behaviour and then making notes on what has been observed retrospectively, whilst a running record involves writing notes about children's behaviour as and when it occurs. Which of these narrative approaches we choose, may depend on whether or not we are involved with the child during the observation (participant observation) or observing from afar (non-participant observation). A running record is more suited to nonparticipant observation as not being directly involved in the play activity, enables us to observe carefully, making discreet notes without distracting or influencing the child's behaviour. Sheridan was likely to have been engaged with the children she observed in her professional medical capacity and so would probably have written diarized notes after the event.

Diary methods can be challenging as they require accurate recall of events. To minimize this issue, it is important to write entries as soon as possible. Running records can be challenging as they occur in real time. This means we need to make on the spot decisions about what to note down and how much detail to provide. This can be managed by limiting the time spent observing and deciding, where possible, what types of things will be noted. Developing a personal form of shorthand can also be useful.

Examples of a diary entries and a running record, based on children interacting with building blocks are provided below. We can see how the child of six months spends time exploring the sensory properties of the blocks (mouthing them and banging them together and against the table). At 15 months, the child begins to explore what they can do with the blocks, balancing them on top of each other to make a tower.

Example 1: A diary entry

Child: Ellie

Age: 6 months

Context: In the nursery on the carpet area

Present: JH (observer) and Ellie (other children proximal but not present)

Date: 10.6.16

I took Ellie over to the carpet area. The wooden bricks were out of their box, spread out over the mat. I laid Ellie on the carpet on her tummy. She is able to lift her head and balance on her arms to support herself. She immediately reached for a brick, bringing it straight to her mouth. She sucked and mouthed it before releasing it so it fell to the floor. She looked at the bricks momentarily before reaching for another. She repeated her actions, mouthing the brick with her lips and tongue. I sat Ellie up. She picked up another brick so that she had one in each hand. She mouthed both before knocking them together to make a banging sound. She looked at me (I think surprised at the noise). She knocked the bricks together a further few times.

Notes:

Ellie seemed really interested in the corners of the bricks, as if she noticed a difference in how these felt on her tongue compared with the flat surfaces. I also wondered if Ellie actually meant to release the brick from grasp or whether her grip just loosened, I couldn't tell if it was done on purpose or not.

Example 2: Running record

Child: James

Age: 15 months

Context: At a low table in the construction corner of the nursery

Present: James (other children proximal but not present)

Date: 12.6.16

Time	Notes
12.00	James walks quickly over to the construction area. There are no other children present and he seems attracted to the wooden bricks, which have been placed onto a low table.
12.05	James moves the bricks around with his arm in a sweeping action, shuffling them around from side to side. He is saying 'lalalala' as he does this, there is noise from a table nearby but he is not distracted.
12.08	He picks up individual bricks and bangs them on the table, firstly with one hand and then with one in each hand. He bangs them harder and harder making a louder and louder sound. He closes his eyes as if startling himself with the noise he is making. This continues for a full minute, changing to different bricks but repeating the same banging action.
12.10	James's focus is now on stacking the bricks. He picks one up and tries to balance it on top of another. It falls and he picks it up and repositions it. He takes another and places this one very gently on the top of the others. He pokes the tower and it topples over. He begins to rebuild it but after placing one brick, is distracted by a group of children playing in the sand.
12.13	James moves to the sand area. Block play ends.

Notes:

James seemed really engaged and absorbed with the bricks. There was quite a lot of noise from the sand and he wasn't distracted at all, paying full attention for quite a few minutes.

The extent to which we are able to generalize from our observations depends on whether our sample is representative and whether our findings are likely to be replicated on different occasions and in different contexts. In chapter 1, Sheridan describes how different types of play emerge in developmental sequence. In chapter 3, she describes key milestones in children's development, noting changes in social, cognitive, language and physical abilities. These accounts would have emerged from her extensive observations of children's play over time, where patterns in behaviour amongst children of similar ages were noted. Sheridan's conclusions about how children's play evolves over time, and both reflects and supports their development, is based on the collective consideration of her extensive data set.

One difficulty associated with the narrative approaches outlined above is deciding exactly what to note down and how much detail to provide. Narrative approaches are often best suited to short observations of sole children and as such, it can take time to develop a large enough data set from which we can make inferences about patterns in children's behaviour. Sheridan would have conducted numerous observations of children of various ages in her practice to inform her ideas over a considerable time scale. This is not always practical.

Some of these issues can be overcome by developing specific observation schedules suitable for use with groups of children that are structured to capture what children are doing at certain intervals in a particular time period (time sampling) or when instances of a specific behaviour are observed (event sampling). This allows us to systematically gather data in a form that could be replicated by others. It also allows us to capture larger data sets in a shorter time frame. There is much flexibility in structured observation schedules and they can be designed and adapted to suit multiple needs. They can be used to gather basic frequency data or relatively rich narrative description.

A sampling method used to investigate how children of different ages play with building blocks is provided below.

Example 3: Sampling technique

Date: 19.6.16

Context: Bricks are placed on a low table in the corner of the construction area

Aim: To observe how children of different ages in the nursery use the bricks

Observation period: 10.30am – 12.30pm (notes made whenever a child visits the area during this period)

Observer: JH

Time	Child	Age	Others	Details	Notes
2 min	DM	15m	/	Alone, wandered to table, picked up bricks with both hands and put both to mouth, banged them on table and then together. Repeated.	Largely distracted, not engaged
5 min	CF	3:3	HG alongside	CF ran over to the bricks and gathered up a large pile from around the table in front of herself. HG arrived and CF looked over. CF built towers of different colours up to five bricks high and passed some bricks over the HG. She made similar towers.	Some signs of social play, giving some bricks to HG as if knowing they should share
7 min	GH	3:4	PP interacts	GH arrived at the table and immediately began to make what looked like a building with the bricks. PP arrived and said let's make a road. They lined up bricks either side to make what looked like a roadway. GH took a brick and 'drove' it (with car noise). PP copied with a further brick. This continued for several minutes with lots of bricks being 'driven' and 'parked' at the end of the road.	Lots of interaction, shared ideas, laughing and smiling

Time	Child	Age	Others	Details	Notes
2 min	SP	12m	/	SP has just started to walk and carefully toddled to the low table. She looked at the bricks for a while, balancing herself on the table edge before lifting one hand to reach for a brick. It was brought to her mouth and she sucked it while looking over at the other bricks. She tried to take another with the other hand, this left her unsupported and she wobbled. She sat down with the single brick to mouth it further before releasing it and leaving the area.	Play seemed disrupted when SP wobbled, letting go of the table edge
6 min	FF	2:9	/	FF engaged with the bricks for considerable time. They were sorted into colours and shapes before being used to make a long 'train like' model. She pushed the long model from one side of the table to the other and back. She placed bricks on top of the long model and pushed it from side to side again but the added bricks fell down. She didn't replace them but reverted back to her original game.	Play ended when time for lunch was called. I think she would have continued to play, she was very engaged.

From this, we can see how younger children spend time playing with the blocks for a shorter time periods, using them to make noise or balancing them into towers. They mainly play alone. Older children play with the blocks for longer in more elaborate ways, showing some signs of interacting with others. They use the blocks to make models, which they sometimes narrate. To get a clear picture of age differences in children's block play, this process could be completed on numerous occasions. Findings could be grouped into those relating to children of different ages, and similarities and differences noted. Separate columns for making notes in relation to different developmental domains could also be added (e.g. reflections on social, cognitive, physical or language skills that are observed).

Summary

■ Systematic observations of children's play have allowed us to track how play skills evolve over time to both support and reflect development.

■ Observations of children's play provides a useful insight into their behaviour across developmental domains.

■ As children's natural mode of action, play is a useful environment for observing children's health and development as it is likely to best reflect their skills and abilities.

■ Key skills in successful observation include being accurate, objective and systematic.

Give yourself some time to think

■ Try and locate some images that depict preformationism. They provide a real insight into beliefs about human development during this period.

■ Practice your own observation skills. Use some of the techniques detailed here (for example, the diary method or a structured observation schedule). What are the strengths and limitations of the approaches you used? How objective were you when recording your observations? Were your observations recorded accurately?

■ Source one or two of the standardized observation methods detailed in this chapter (e.g. PIPPS, POS). Do you think these might be useful for your practice?

Useful reading

Bellmann, M., Lungain, S. and Ankett, A. (1996). *Schedule of growing skills*. London: NFER-Nelson.

Epstein, A. S., Schweinhart, L. J., DeBruin-Parecki, A., & Robin, K. B. (2004). 'Preschool assessment: A guide to developing a balanced approach.' *Preschool Policy Matters* 7, 1–2.

Hamilton, G. (2016). Honouring Dr. Mary D. Sheridan. The Royal Society of Medicine Wall of Honour. Available online at www.rsm-wallofhonour.com (accessed 29 June 2016).

Howard, J. & McInnes, K. (2013). *The essence of play: A practice companion for professionals working with children and young people*. London: Routledge.

Lorch, M., & Hellal, P. (2010). Darwin's 'Natural Science of Babies'. *Journal of the History of the Neurosciences* 19(2), 140–57.

Sharman, C., Cross, W. and Vennis, D. (2007). *Observing Children and Young People*, 4th ed. London: Continuum.

Sheridan, M. (1978). *STYCAR developmental sequences*. Windsor, Ontario: NFER Publishing Company Ltd.

3

The development of children's play: Sheridan's observations

This chapter presents Sheridan's *original observations* of the ages and stages at which significant manifestations of behaviour usually appear, supporting the development of children's repertoire of play skills. Understanding children's development can help us to make the best provision for their play. However, it is important to bear in mind that wide variations are to be expected. The chapter describes children's development in age-defined sections; however, the ages provided should be taken only as a guide and they are not necessarily the earliest or latest points at which a behaviour might appear. This variation is evident in the illustrations used by Sheridan to exemplify her observations where sometimes the age of the child pictured does not match the age with which the section is principally concerned. Of particular importance is the growth of children's ability to play and how their acquired play skills feed into further development. Note how Sheridan has captured the fine detail associated with children's behaviour across developmental domains within the illustrations. These line drawings are a defining feature of Sheridan's work. Photographs of children engaged in similar behaviours to those depicted by Sheridan in other chapters of the book demonstrate the currency of her original observations.

The specific aims of this chapter are:

- To highlight the value of Sheridan's real-world observations in documenting children's development in play.

- To encourage readers, in light of the depth and detail presented by Sheridan, to reflect on their own observation skills and to practice some of the observational techniques outlined in chapter 2.

The newborn quickly learns to attract and welcome the attention of primary caregivers who are usually their first playmates. Although vigorous movements, smiles and coos indicate baby's response to enjoyable stimulation, behaviour becomes more purposeful over the coming months and is no longer merely a manifestation of stimulus and response but increasingly a question of selective sensory intake (reception), which is then processed within the brain (interpretation) and results in some appropriate motor outcome (expression).

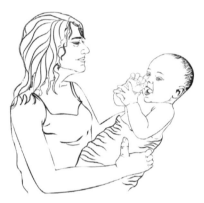

6 weeks: Caregivers are usually the first playmates and lively interchange involves looking, listening, vocalizing and body movements.

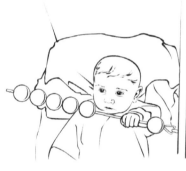

10 weeks: Baby can grasp the bar and focus on a coloured ball, but is not yet able to co-ordinate hand and eyes.

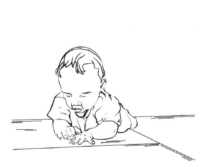

12 weeks: Lying on their front, they scratch at the table cover, enjoying simultaneous sight and sound.

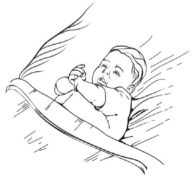

3 months: With head and back well supported baby demonstrates good hand–eye co-ordination in finger-play.

Hand–eye co-ordination is demonstrated at about 10–12 weeks when a recumbent child deliberately brings their hands together over the upper chest and engages in finger-play. About the same time, when lying on their stomach holding the head and shoulders up steadily, they will open and shut their hands to scratch the surface where they lie, with some appreciation of the simultaneous production of sight and sound. A handheld toy (such as a rattle) can be clasped and brought towards the face, but sometimes baby may bash their chin and any glances made at it are fleeting.

By about 14 weeks, baby develops increased control over head, neck and eye muscles simultaneously to hand grasp, and can hold the toy and steadily regard it. At about 18–20 weeks they can reach for and grasp an offered rattle, look at it with prolonged gaze and shake it. They can clasp and unclasp objects alternately and bring objects towards and away from the mouth.

By 6 months, muscular control, vision and hand–eye co-ordination are so advanced that baby can reach for and seize any nearby object. They have not yet developed voluntary hand release. They discover their feet and often use them as auxiliary claspers. Every grasped object is brought to the mouth. They are beginning to comprehend the permanence of people but not yet the permanence of things. When a toy falls from their hand, unless it is within their range of vision, it ceases to exist.

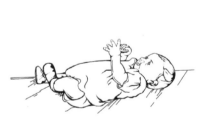 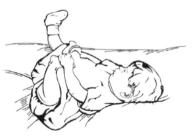

4½ months: With consistent hand–eye co-ordination, baby holds the teething ring between their hands, opening and closing them alternately.

5½ months: Baby discovers their feet and reaches out to them, demonstrating foot, hand and eye co-ordination.

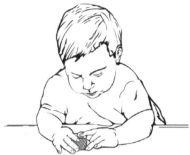

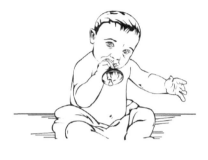

6 months: With high concentration, baby makes characteristic age-related two-handed approach to a block.

6 months: A bell is grasped with both hands, the bell is transferred to one hand and then brought to the mouth.

■ Develops a strong bond with responsive primary caregiver.

■ Hand–eye co-ordination improves and movements become more controlled and purposeful.

■ Objects are brought to the mouth for exploration.

■ Begins to understand the permanence of people but not objects.

6-12 months

At about 7 months, the baby is able to pass a toy from one hand to the other with voluntary hand release. From about 8 months, the baby can sit steadily on the floor, stretch out in all directions for toys within reach without falling over, and is able to reach towards eye-catching objects.

From 9 months, babies usually first regard a new toy appraisingly for a few moments, as if to judge its qualities, before reaching for it, and they enjoy manipulating one toy at a time. A little later, from imitation or discovery, they can combine two objects in some active way, such as banging a couple of wooden spoons together or rattling a spoon in a cup. During this time, baby is beginning to develop an ability to differentiate between familiar people and unfamiliar strangers. Object permanence develops around 9–10 months, as baby will lift a cushion to look underneath it for a half-hidden play object. It is not long after that a developed ability exists to detect a hidden object. During this time, babies enjoy producing the

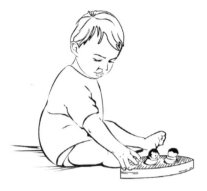

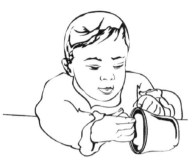

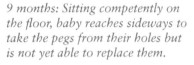

9 months: Sitting competently on the floor, baby reaches sideways to take the pegs from their holes but is not yet able to replace them.

9 months: Although not yet able to release the blocks into the cup, baby has some notion of the nature of the container and keeps on trying.

simultaneous noise and tactile sensation of banging or sliding solid objects. All babies, as they become more mobile, increasingly seek proximity to their primary caregiver partly for the reassurance of constant availability and partly to seek co-operation in play.

From 9–12 months, babies begin to understand the import of the primary caregiver's spoken communications: first the cadences of vocal intonation, then of a few single-word forms and eventually of the simply phrased instructions and boundaries in recurrent

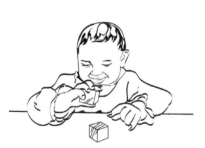

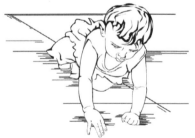

9 months: Having watched a playmate build a tower of blocks to knock over, baby tries to imitate. Grasping right hand and pointing left index finger are well shown.

10 months: Creeping towards an eye-catching plaything and reaching for it.

situational contexts. Babies begin to find meaning in their homely world and like to watch and listen to familiar adults, be touched, talked to and played with. The attention, relationships and play of the baby are still engaged and satisfied mainly at the level of ongoing perceptions, but immediate, brief imitations indicate the possession of a short-term memory and baby proceeds with the establishment of a long-term memory-bank. For the latter, all sorts of memories become stored, related to significant somatic, cognitive and affective experiences, for the purpose of instantaneous recognition, retrieval and creative assembly when needed.

Early play remains repetitive unless the primary caregiver indicates the next step. In these homely ways, a child learns during the first year that things keep their properties even in movement, but the behaviour of people tends to be unpredictable. Babies must be able to move about their familiar world so as to acquire a working knowledge of its nature and its possibilities while learning to control their own behaviours and relationships within it, before they can communicate wishes, attitudes and intentions with regard to it. Babies are also able to recognize situational constancy in home surroundings. For instance, they know when the primary caregiver is out of sight for a short time, and they begin to tolerate extended intervals of time and space between themselves and the primary caregiver.

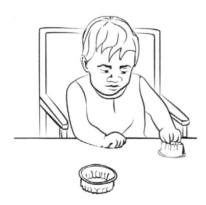

10 months: Enjoying the simultaneous sight and sound made by sliding plastic pastry cutters on the table.

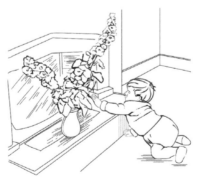

11 months: Having acquired the ability to crawl, baby explores their environment.

At home, babies balance a need for close proximity to the primary caregiver with a need to explore, nicely integrating motor activity with sensory alertness and emotional satisfaction. In the first 12 months baby has already travelled a far distance from early dominance by neonatal reflexes, to present individualistic manifestations of capability and personality. To achieve full potential baby must be supported to travel even further and more rapidly during the next couple of years.

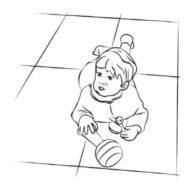

11 months: Baby improves their skill in locomotion by carrying two objects simultaneously.

- Acquires hand-release skill and can now pass objects from hand to hand and drop things voluntarily.

- Understands the permanence of objects.

- Can tolerate short intervals of time away from the primary caregiver but will seek proximity for reassurance and co-operation in play.

- Begins to manipulate individual objects.

- Some brief imitative behaviour begins to emerge and baby will enjoy banging, rattling and sliding solid objects.

12-18 months

In this period children become increasingly mobile, inquisitive and wilful. They have an increased ability to attend to detail and a growing recognition of cause and effect. The child is no longer satisfied with mainly perceptual phenomena and quickly loses interest in events which are presented mainly as distant, repetitive or unrewarding. This understanding is first manifest through their own experiences, and actions. The child is dominated by an urge to explore and exploit the surrounding environment: for example, when exploring cupboards, to manipulate, smell and taste the objects within, sometimes presenting them to the primary caregiver. Children at this stage are also able to manipulate blocks with a good pincer grasp.

Percussion tools are still employed to experiment in the synchronization of sound and strike; and with increasing skill in upright ambulation and navigation, the child is able to push and pull large wheeled toys and guide small ones by hand or on the end of a string. Young children during this period are still tied to everyday family realities where role play features in short episodes. They also begin

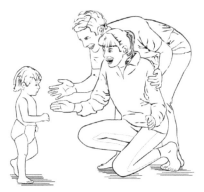

11 months: First steps require caregiver encouragement and considerable courage.

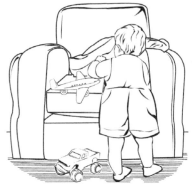

12 months: Holding on to the furniture and stepping sideways, they cruise about the room, investigating objects of interest.

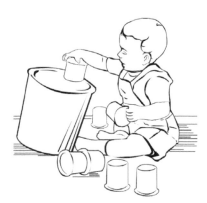

14 months: Having gained some appreciation of the phenomenon of container and contained, they greatly enjoy putting objects in and out of the wastepaper bin.

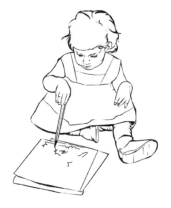

12 months: Holds the pencil in an age-typical fashion. A few moments later the pencil was shifted to the other hand.

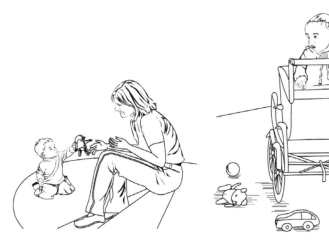

12 months: This give-and-take play involved not only playthings but linguistic interchange.

12 months: Having thrown out all the playthings, they call loudly to get them back.

to communicate needs and feelings quite effectively in a medley of large expressive gestures, loud, tuneful vocalizations and a small but ever-increasing repertoire of single words, while showing a growing interest in naming objects and pictures, in repeating words and in listening to people talking.

At this developmental stage of limited cognitive, social and language appreciation, a doll or animal toy is treated like any other plaything. For the child, objects hold no true emotional significance, owing to immature preoccupation with the 'me' and only very primitive realization of the 'not me'. Consequently, so far as the child is concerned, young babies (who do not 'intend' anything) are not personalities in their own right, but merely objects. Social learning is undoubtedly entirely ego-centred at first: that is, 'self-tied', rather than 'self-ish'. Acceptable externalized or 'detached-from-self' activities, leading later to the practice of unselfishness, sharing, taking turns and eventually to compassionate behaviour, do not, indeed cannot, develop until a child has learned first the primary distinction of 'me' and 'not me', then the distinction of 'me' and 'you', and finally the distinction of 'us' and 'them', which is the keystone of social communication. Some of this learning depends upon appreciation of what is 'mine' and what is 'not mine', and of what is 'yours' and 'theirs'.

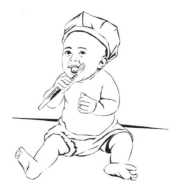 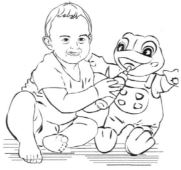 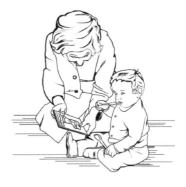

12 months: They cannot yet name these objects but they are well able to demonstrate their use in relation to the self.

12 months: Shows a vague notion of the objects' application outside of the self.

12 months: This interest in books is greatly encouraged by the caregiver.'

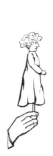 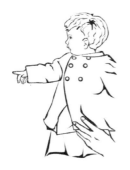 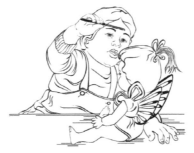

13 months: The puppet evokes delighted pointing and loud vocalization.

15 months: They now clearly understand the functions of a comb and speak a recognizable version of the word.

Until this final stage of cognitive and emotive maturation has been reached, the child's egocentricity leads to the unshakeable conviction that all things rightfully belong to the child. As soon as children are mobile they should be provided with some playthings and a place (for territory) so that they may learn not only the satisfactions but the accepted conventions of personal and territorial possession, including the need to respect the rights of others.

Key observations

■ Increased mobility widens opportunities for exploration.

■ There is less repetitive action and increasing attention to object detail.

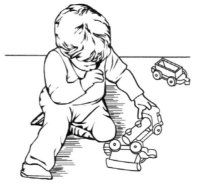

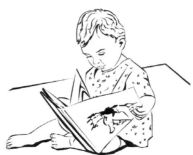

They cannot quite link up these train carriages.

Squatting on the floor, they study the picture book with interest, but turn several pages at a time.

- ■ Enjoyment of push-and-pull toys indicates some recognition of cause and effect.

- ■ Can communicate needs and wishes using an increasing repertoire of words and gestures.

- ■ Remains relatively egocentric and unable to separate 'me' from 'not me'.

18-24 months

Between 18 and 24 months, with rapidly improving control of the body and limbs, a child engages in many gross-motor activities such as pushing, pulling and carrying large objects, as well as climbing on furniture, low walls and steps. Sitting on a small tricycle, the child can steer it on course, but propels it forward with feet on the ground. A sense of danger, like understanding and use of language, is still very limited. However, a desire for independent action is boundless. Therefore, the child requires constant supervision to be protected from danger.

The child becomes increasingly interested in the nature and detailed exploitation of small objects, constantly practising and refining manipulative abilities. Young children will play contentedly at floor level for prolonged periods with suitable, durable toys, provided they know that a familiar and attentive adult is near. The child will enjoy putting small toys in and out of containers and is able to build towers of blocks, varying from 3 at 18 months to 6 or more at 2 years. Children are able to experiment for lengthening periods of time with water and sand, or malleable materials like clay and dough, using their hands and simple tools effectively, but as yet without the ability to plan or achieve an end-product.

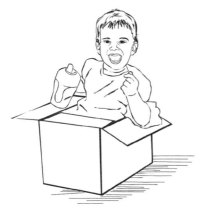

20 months: An irresistible urge to get in and out of large boxes, perhaps learning their relative size and position.

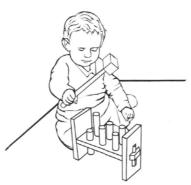

20 months: Enjoys the simultaneous sight and sound and muscular precision of the hammering activity.

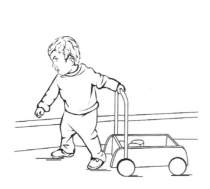

18 months: They walk backwards and sideways, pulling and steering a trolley containing a collection of bricks.

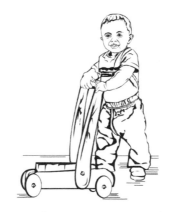

18 months: Discovering control of a push-and-pull toy.

Drawings have no real pictorial representation and although one hand is tending to show dominance, such preference is still very variable; the child continues to use either hand freely and sometimes both together. These manifestations of unequal, shifting or perhaps non-simultaneous appreciation and control of laterality continue with decreasing frequency throughout the preschool years.

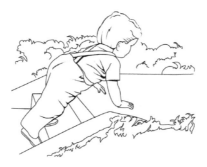

18 months: Crawling swiftly up the garden steps. (The usual sequence of movements – right hand, left foot; left hand, right foot – is clearly shown.)

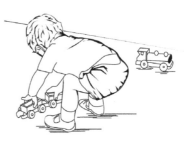

18 months: Playing with the same toys as three months earlier, they are now able to link the train carriages.

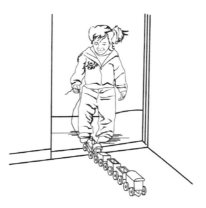

2 years: Having successfully linked up the trucks, they pull the whole train through the doorway, walking backwards and round the corner.

The child is still egocentric but is actively building memories from mimicking the behaviours of those around them. Role play and situational 'pretend' play, which are characteristic of this stage, might involve the child using materials that are readily to hand. For example, nearby cushions and coverings might be used opportunistically while the child plays for a few moments at pretending to go to bed. The child is able to put two or three toys together meaningfully – a doll on a chair; bricks in a truck – but seldom, as yet, makes one object represent another or uses mime to symbolize absent things or events.

From 15–18 months onwards, a child also becomes increasingly interested in picture books, first to recognize and name people, animals, objects and familiar actions (eating and drinking, getting into a car, posting a letter). Soon they can follow a simple story read aloud while exploring the pictures. Next they begin to make comments and ask questions. Some of this love of books and stories, which is very beneficial for language development, is associated with a continued need for close proximity to the primary caregiver, a normal phase of socialization.

By 18 months, the child usually speaks a few single words, such as 'tup' (cup) and 'dink' (drink), in appropriate context as well as a number of meaningful utterances (holophrases) which, to the child, are single words, such as 'gimme' (give me) and 'hee-ya' (here you are); action is linked to what is being said. About 21 months the child begins to put two or more 'real' words together to frame little sentences. These usually refer to very familiar matters, or to needs and happenings in the 'here and now'. The child is now able to

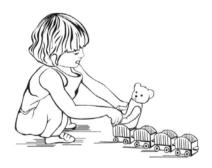

2½ years: Having tried unsuccessfully to step into the train, they are still a little confused regarding the relative size of truck and teddy.

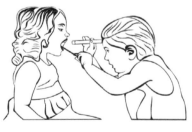

2 years: Medical role play.

communicate effectively wishes, refusal, likes and dislikes through a combination of gestures, and may include a few words and phrases. The child can comprehend most simple language they hear.

Also at about 21 months, children begin to demonstrate their appreciation that miniature (i.e. dolls'-house–size) toys represent things and people in the real world. They clearly show this externalization (or expression) of previously internalized (i.e. memorized) experiences by spontaneously arranging the little toys in meaningful groups, by actively indicating their use in everyday situations, and often by simultaneously talking about them.

Constant sympathetic, but non-stressful adult encouragement to engage in every sort of spontaneous play is essential not only to the contentment but to the fundamental learning of children between 1 and 2 years of age. Through manipulation of playthings, they first discover through their visual, auditory and tactile perceptions what they are and what special properties they possess (i.e. their special quality), then go on to learn what can be done with them (i.e. their special function) and finally how objects can be adapted to suit their own requirements, constructional or make believe (their potentialities). This investigative behaviour is often evident during make-believe play.

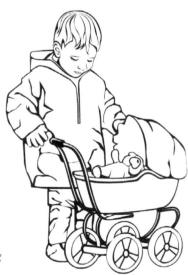

2 years: Imitative role play developing into inventive make believe.

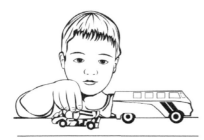

21 months: The beginnings of clearly representative play with miniature toys.

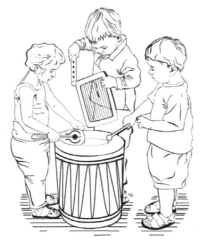

1¾ – 2¼ years: Parallel play using musical instruments in a day nursery.

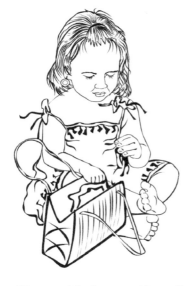

2½ years: The bag provides endless opportunities for exploration, manipulation and imitation.

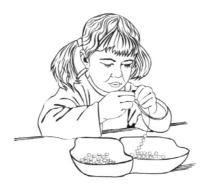

2½ years: Threading beads maintains the child's interest now fingers have acquired sufficient skill.

■ Concentration span increases and desire for independence grows.

■ Now that the child is familiar with objects within their environment, they begin to utilize them in play.

■ There is simple imitative role play of familiar scenes (i.e. mum and baby).

Key observations

- Engages in play with miniature objects but objects are used realistically and not symbolically (i.e. toy bricks might be placed into a toy truck).

- There is a growing interest in print and mark-making activity.

2–3 years

From the age of 2 years, a child is becoming increasingly skilful in every form of motor activity and may be able to ride a tricycle forwards, using the pedals, and steer it round corners. Skills of kicking, throwing and catching a ball increase.

Children's manipulations and constructive skills steadily improve and they are able to hold a pencil halfway down the shaft or near the point, scribbling or imitating to and fro lines and circles on a sheet of paper. The child enjoys simple jigsaw puzzles and can match four or five colours and several shapes.

Children instinctively use a lively form of 'total communication' composed sometimes separately but more often simultaneously of words, gestures, mime and occasionally language codemes. These developments are immediately reflected in their play. The child will still follow familiar adults around the house, imitating and joining in their activities, calling attention to their own efforts, demanding approval, and asking innumerable questions. Extending earlier role play, children invent little make-believe situations, which become

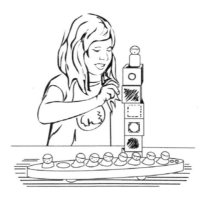

2½ years: Two 'educational toys' being employed for inventive make-believe play. The man is at the top of the lighthouse.

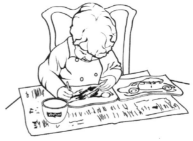

2½ years: Painting at the dining table, indifferent to the fact that the pictures are upside down.

increasingly organized and prolonged, and which they 'play out' with high seriousness. During these mini-dramas they talk aloud to themselves, in appropriate terms, describing and explaining what is being done, instructing themselves with regard to immediately forthcoming actions or formulating their uncertainties. Later they extend their inventions, adding some relevant dialogue to the role play and indicating the beginnings of forward planning, such as collecting suitable items for a dolls' tea party, or materials to construct and drive a make-believe car.

After 2½ years, children's moveable 'self-space' remains chiefly relative to themselves and caregivers, but children are now prepared to admit one or two familiar children briefly into their playworld and to venture intermittently into other children's play. Although they play in close proximity, however, the play itself is mainly of the 'solo' type, so each child needs their own set of playthings and their own piece of 'territory'. At this developmental stage a child seems to realize their physical separateness before appreciating their own cognitive and affective individuality. For some time, therefore, the child remains convinced that the primary caregiver automatically apprehends what the child is feeling, needing and intending. However, under 3 years or so, the child does not expect other children to share the inner workings of their own mind, but assumes their own right to exercise dictatorial behaviour.

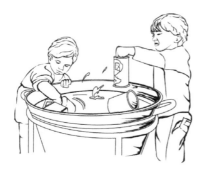

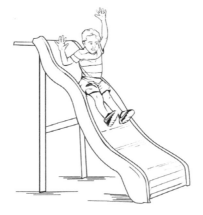

2½–3½ years: Water play in a nursery school, providing an excellent example of parallel play. Each child has their own play materials and play space.

3½ years: Gymnastics on the playground slide.

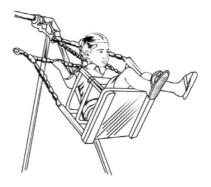

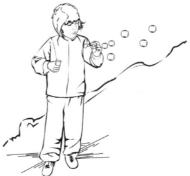

*3 years: The expression is full
of wonder at the changing
appearance of the world beneath
as they swing.*

*3 years: Enjoying the appearance
and behaviour of bubbles.*

Key observations

■ Role play extends to situations reflecting the wider social world (e.g. shopkeeper, doctors and nurses) and some simple narratives may begin to emerge.

■ The child might substitute one object for another in play (i.e. Lego blocks used to represent food in a mealtime scene).

■ The child can match some shapes and colours in a simple jigsaw puzzle.

■ With increased motor control, children will enjoy kicking, throwing and catching a ball.

■ May play in the proximity of other children, but solitary play is predominant and children's own space and materials are important.

■ Pencil control improves and the child may be able to copy simple circular or up-and-down marks.

3-4 years

From 3 years onwards, children still need to play. The child is able to run freely, climb over and about the usual nursery apparatus, negotiate slides, crawl through barrels and jump on small trampolines. The child is able to develop skills in riding a tricycle, confidently using the pedals and steering safely round sharp corners. The child now has a clear appreciation of space in relation to their own body in size and shape, at rest and in movement. The child is able to carry large blocks, planks and boards with the help of co-operative playmates to build constructions in which to conduct a host of vivid make-believe activities.

Hand skills are also rapidly improving through play with small toys like blocks, jigsaw puzzles, miniature cars, dolls' houses and so on, and the child enjoys pencil work and cutting out shapes with scissors. Block building remains popular for many years, proceeding from simple towers to more elaborate structures, ingeniously planned and carefully executed. Children first employ blocks purely as manipulative objects, then through imitation, copying and instruction they gradually extend their forward programming or 'blueprinting' to the construction of structures which (like their spontaneous drawings) they name beforehand. Later, these constructions are often taken into other, more complicated and fanciful play with miniature cars, furniture and dolls to form part of the settings.

From 3 years onwards, puzzles with a greater number of pieces are needed. It is noticeable that many children of this age are more

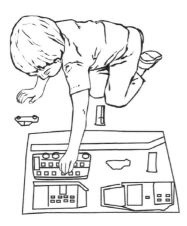

3½ years: Simple insert jigsaw puzzles retain their fascination for much longer than one expects.

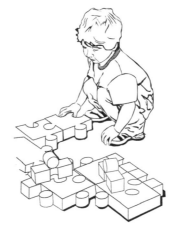

3½ years: They are well able to cope with this more complicated jigsaw puzzle, although its large size necessitated frequent unhurried contemplation.

interested in analytical fitting together of the shapes than building up the picture, so they will construct it from the plain wooden back without regard for the attractively coloured and designed front. Later assembly of a picture with many more pieces becomes all-important. It is not clear why some children perform in this fashion, but it may be that they are manifesting the commonly found sequence of learning which proceeds from general overview, through separate analysis of details, to final immediate synthesis into a well-apprehended whole.

Play with plasticine and other malleable materials can be enjoyable from 3 years onwards, and particularly with over-4s. Spontaneous drawings of 3s and 4s (as distinct from copy-design) become increasingly elaborate and diverse in colour, form and content, although they still remain chiefly concerned with people, houses, vehicles and flowers. The 3-year-old does not name the drawing until it is finished. Then, about 4 years, the child will announce beforehand what is about to be drawn, indicating some sort of preliminary 'blueprint' in thinking prior to beginning. By 4–4½ years, children may be expected to engage amicably in all sorts of self-directed play activities with peers. At this stage, improvised constructional building, table and floor games, dressing up and make-believe play are greatly favoured. Children need opportunities through play for discussion, planning, sharing, taking turns and recognition of agreed rules.

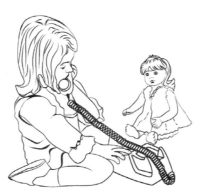

3 years: Supremely secure, engaging in elaborate role make-believe play.

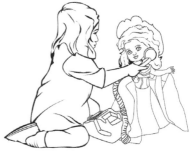

3 years: There are two participants and in the dialogue, using different tones of voice and choice of words.

Interest in music-making, usually in the form of percussion instruments or simple wind instruments, often begins to show itself from 3½ to 4 years. Children can manifest unusually sophisticated tastes very early, not only in their listening, but in expression, recognizing and recalling tunes learned from adults and older children, or heard on the radio. Some may ask for and even manage to play such musical instruments as are within their capacity to manipulate. Meanwhile, between 3 and 4 years a child's ability to use spoken

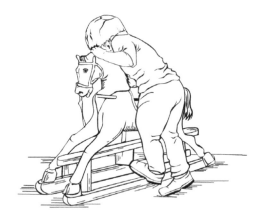

3½ years: Gracefully mounting a large, old rocking horse.

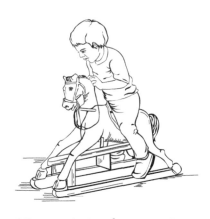

3½ years: Active play merges into make-believe show jumping.

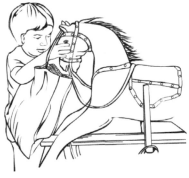

3½ years: After the show jumping, the horse is fondly fed from a shopping bag.

language rapidly improves both in vocabulary and syntax so that, in spite of residual infantile mispronunciations and grammatical errors, speech is generally intelligible even to people outside the immediate family. Children and their playmates informally communicate in a glorious mixture of words, exaggerated vocal cadences, facial expressions and telling gestures, and they understand each other perfectly.

By 4 years, verbal interchanges of every sort – friendly, informative, questioning, argumentative, explanatory and instructive – become increasingly evident in all aspects of play, especially in make-believe

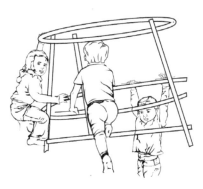

2½–4 years: Children enjoying active play in the park with their caregivers near by.

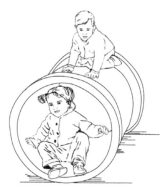

2½–4 years: Young children in an adventure playground, demonstrating several interesting aspects of activity play.

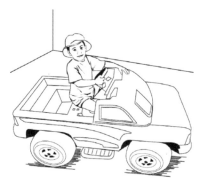

3½ years: Demonstrating skilful motor control and excellent spatial sense.

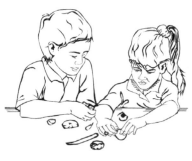

3 and 3½ years: Children making small plasticine models of domestic and other objects.

situations. Once free communication has been established within any group, the signs of leadership show up clearly, with the dominant child deciding who shall play the major roles and who shall be the subsidiary characters. The leader may or may not generously agree to later interchanges of roles and taking turns. At this stage children's make-believe and subjective worlds can be so vivid to themselves that what is fact and what is fiction can become hazy; inexperienced caregivers may be startled by apparent blatant disregard for objective truth. Four-year-olds delight in rhymes, riddles, simple jokes and verbal teasing. They love having stories read to them, especially when they can simultaneously look at illustrations. Although they now appreciate peers to play with, they still enjoy being with their parents and siblings at home, continuing to learn by imitating, trying out new skills, listening, talking and asking endless questions.

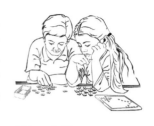

3½ and 5½ years: Managing a very complicated jigsaw puzzle, carefully explaining their strategies.

By this time, the child can mentally detach the physical aspects of 'self' from those of 'non-self' sufficiently well to be able to envisage the situation of hills, houses, bridges and other prominent features in the landscape from another's position in space, and they can appreciate some of the implications of visual perspective, although this does not yet appear in their drawings. They also begin

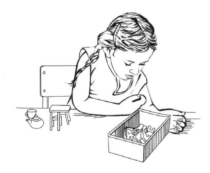

4½ years: Handed a box of miniature toys, the child scrutinizes the collection in situ before selecting items for assembly. A younger child would probably first spread them all out on the table-top.

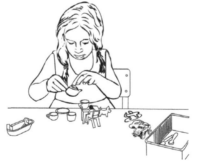

A few minutes later, assembly is almost complete: domestic items together, bath 'upstairs' and items of transport 'outside'.

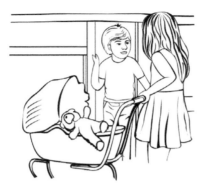

3½ and 5 years: Elaborate make-believe house play.

to demonstrate a growing sense of compassion and responsibility. Appetite for adventure is not always matched by appreciation of the dangers: children enjoy taking risks that end in self-discovered boundaries!

Key observations

■ Children now enjoy playing with similar-aged peers.

■ Role play and make believe become increasingly imaginative and complex.

■ In a small social group, children learn to negotiate roles, to share and take turns.

■ Increased mastery of language allows children to delight in simple jokes and rhymes.

■ There is a clear appreciation of body size and shape and the child can run freely, climb, crawl and jump.

■ Advanced fine motor skill facilitates more detailed drawing, and children may be able to cut out simple shapes using scissors.

■ Children will enjoy the process of making things, using, for example, dough or building blocks, or gluing and sticking.

From this stage onwards, the child steadily continues to develop everyday competence and powers of communication. In play they show an increasing enjoyment not only of elaborate make-believe activities but of complicated indoor and outdoor games which require knowledgeable preliminary instruction, hard practice, strict adherence to rules and a sense of fair play. Personal aptitudes for sports, crafts and the creative arts become ever more apparent in the child's selective use of leisure time, choice of companions and the games they play, whether at home, in playgrounds with special equipment, or in open fields and streets with no equipment at

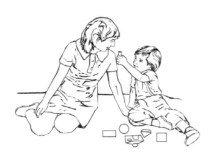

4½ years: Coloured plastic shapes provide excellent opportunities for inventive picture-making and conversation.

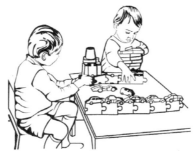

4½ and 5 years: At playgroup, the children collaborate in constructing an elaborate street scene complete with church, high-rise flats, flyover and traffic.

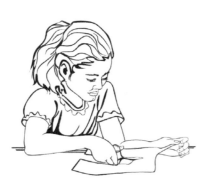

4½ years: Cutting out a carpet for the dolls' house.

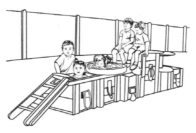

3–5 years: Children attending a day nursery. This elaborate construction, assembled and dismantled every day, provides opportunity for every kind of outdoor play.

all other than the chants and rituals of long-unwritten tradition, coupled with lively contemporary improvisations.

For the next few years the separate interests of boys and girls are clearly evident in their spontaneous play, although in school playgrounds teachers usually organize and encourage mixed-play activities.

Key observations

■ Children steadily continue to develop everyday competence and powers of communication.

■ There is an increasing enjoyment of more structured, rule-based games.

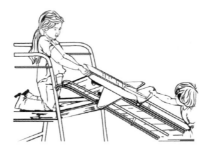

3½ and 5 years: Co-operative activity play on the slide.

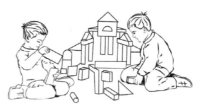

4 years: Elaborate building with large wooden blocks involving considerable forward planning and precise construction.

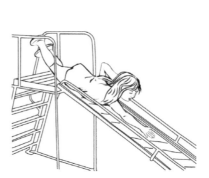

5 years: Child on a slide.

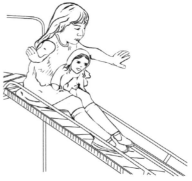

5 years: Gymnastics on the slide, involving appropriate verbal instruction of the doll.

- Increased improvisational ability means play often needs minimal props and good use can be made of open-ended materials.

- Personal aptitudes for sports, crafts and the creative arts become ever more apparent.

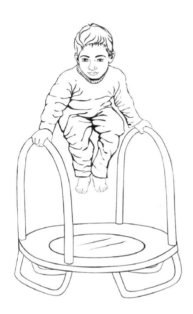

4½ years: A competent performer on the trampoline.

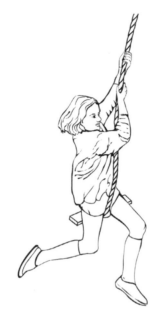

A certain element of danger adds to the attraction of this swing.

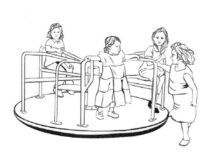

A group of familiar friends on the roundabout in the park.

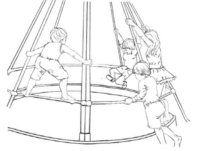

The same children performing skilfully on a more difficult roundabout (they call it 'doing Olympics').

Summary

Sheridan's observations document how, as children grow, they develop new competencies that contribute to their *ability to play* in different ways. Using the secure base formed through attachment with the primary caregiver, they explore the environment, at first using their senses. Through continued interaction with others, they gradually develop communication and social skills, recognizing a world outside of the self. With mobility and dexterity, they explore objects and their properties, utilizing them in increasingly complex ways. Through this expanding repertoire of play behaviour, children learn about themselves, about others and about the world around them, *developing through play*. Beginning with early sensory experiences, through the controlled manipulation and symbolic use of objects, to imaginative make believe, children's progressive play skills offer them unique ways to experience and make sense of their world (Jennings, 1999). The pattern of 'What is this?', 'What does this do?', 'What *can* I do with this?' and 'What *could* I do with this?' is evident in possibility thinking across the lifespan (Craft, 2005).

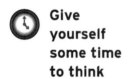

Give yourself some time to think

- Spend some time considering how Sheridan's observations map on to the developmental sequences of Piaget, Parten and Erikson (described in chapter 1).

  – What do you think are the notable advances in social, cognitive and emotional development?

- Observe a child or group of children at play.

  – How easy did you find the observation process?

- How did you decide what to observe and how to record the information?

- How do your observations fit with Sheridan's in relation to observed competencies and the child/children's age(s)?

Useful reading

Howard, J., & McInnes, K. (2013a). *The essence of play.* London: Routledge.

Hughes, F. (2010). *Children, play and development,* 4th Edition. London: SAGE.

Smidt, S. (2015). *Observing young children: The role of observation and assessment in early childhood settings.* London: Routledge.

Outlines of some particular play sequences

4

The previous chapter presented Sheridan's original observations of children's play. Through her observations, Sheridan illustrated how play changes with age as children gradually acquire new competencies that both reflect and influence their development. We saw how play progresses from that which is sensory in nature, to symbolic play, imaginative play and play that incorporates rules. Sheridan also detailed the increasingly social nature of play.

To exemplify the changes she had noted in children's play over time, Sheridan selected observations of children using particular materials and grouped these together in 'play sequences'. We present these sequences here. As in chapter 2, the ages noted below each illustration represent the child's age at the time of Sheridan's observation and are not necessarily indicative of the earliest or latest time at which behaviours might emerge. Also remain mindful that wide variation is to be expected.

The specific aims of this chapter are:

- To outline some particular play sequences involving cup, bell and block play, mark making and small world activity.

- To highlight, by showing children of different ages interacting with the same materials, the ways in which play changes over time.

- To provide a brief summary of each play sequence with reference to theories of play and child development.

Cup play

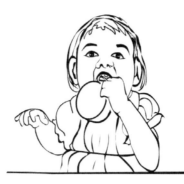

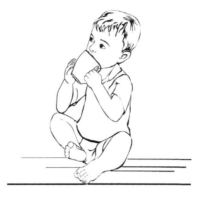

6 months: Having grasped with both hands, baby passes to one hand and brings the most prominent feature of the cup to the mouth.

9 months: Grasping the cup right side up with both hands, baby brings the rim to their mouth, looking at the caregiver.

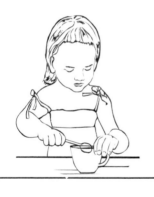

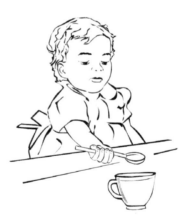

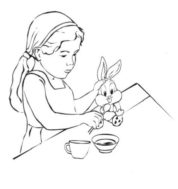

12 months: Having just observed me place cup and spoon on table after testing their hearing by stroking the rim of this cup, they seize the cup and spoon and successfully imitate.

12 months: The foregoing imitation reminds them of the true function of cups and spoons and they promptly offer a clear example of definition-by-use.

2½ years: Cups, spoons and other related domestic items are happily incorporated into make-believe play.

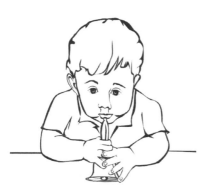

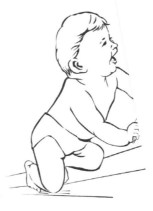

*24 weeks: Grasps bell at base
with both hands, obviously
concentrating serious attention on
activity. Immediately afterwards
the top of the handle is brought to
the mouth.*

*9 months: Grasps mid-handl
one hand and delightedly ba
noisily and repeatedly on tab*

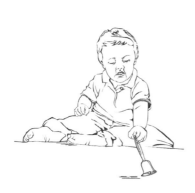

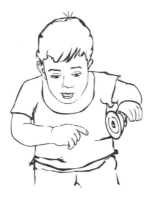

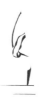

Block

*10 months: Seizes top of
handle with one hand and
rings bell, enjoying musical
sound.*

*11 months: Pokes at clapper
with index finger.*

*12 mont
reminds
act accor
decide wh
exploratio
definition-*

In these sequences of cup and bell play, we can see clear progression in the infants' exploration of materials, using their hands and mouths to understand an objects properties. This sensory exploration of objects is consistent with the Embodied play described by Jennings (1999) and the sensory play of Piaget (1951). Here, children explore the world around them through sight, sound, touch and taste. We gradually begin to see the initial stages of pretend play emerging, where the child uses objects in their play. In the cup example the object is used in a way that is consistent with its realistic function. In the case of the bell play however, pretend play ability is more complex and the bell is used as if it were a cup. As Sheridan notes, this may have been fortuitous exploration, however, it could also signal the appearance of symbolism, where one object can be used in pretend play to represent another (Piaget, 1951). At 12 months, these sequences demonstrate the child's ability to imitate action, a skill Sheridan associated with children of around seven months of age. The ability to imitate has been the focus of much research in developmental science and findings demonstrate that the nature and accuracy of imitation develops of over time (Meltzoff et al., 2013). There is increasing evidence to suggest however, that even as early as 12–20 days old, babies are able to imitate facial expressions (Meltzoff & Moor, 1997).

play

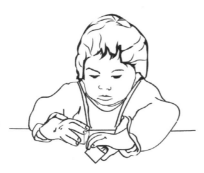

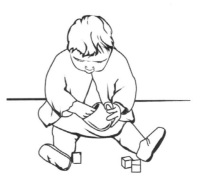

9 months: Holding a block competently in each hand, they bring them together in interested comparison. A few moments later the child found considerable pleasure in clicking them together.

12 months: Having found a block hidden under the cup, the child begins to explore some further possibilities on their own account.

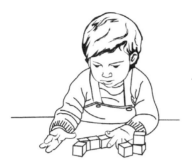

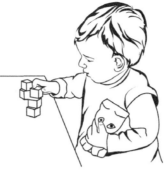

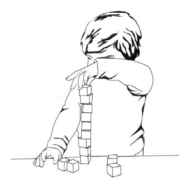

15 months: Blocks are arranged as shown entirely by the child. They seem to be recalling some previous game of 'pushing a train' with an older playmate.

15 months: The child has always enjoyed handling blocks and readily builds little towers of two or three with their right hand while grasping a larger stuffed animal toy with the left.

2 years: A particularly competent young architect. Having built half the tower with their right hand, they shift attention to the left. This interesting form of self-training is very common.

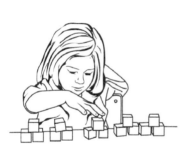

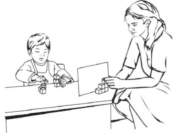

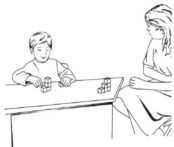

3 years: A fine example of previous learning using up every block to form a bridge and counting them aloud.

3½ years: The caregiver is building three steps out of bricks behind a screen for the child to copy – a relatively complex task for a child at this age.

3½ years: But with long experience of constructive block play the child has no difficulty in copying the model.

As well as highlighting the same progression through the sensory exploration of objects as exemplified in the cup and bell sequences, in the case of block play we are able to see how the child extends their understanding of the object properties by banging the two bricks together. The child is learning about cause and effect and the way in which they are able to impact on their environment (Goswami, 2014). Piaget (1951) made a similar observation of

Summary – block play

cause and effect with his own child. He noted how they kicked the cot mobile, first by mistake and then, with intention as they realized they were able to make it move. The second part of this sequence is also of significance, where the child seeks out the brick that has been hidden underneath a cup. Seeking out an object that is hidden from view demonstrates that the child has 'object permanence' and understands that something exists even when it goes out of sight. At 12 months old, this child's behaviour is consistent with the age at which Piaget (1951) considered the early stages of object permanence would appear. Further research, however, has demonstrated that children exhibit signs of object permanence as early as three months old (Baillargeon & DeVos, 1991).

Mark making

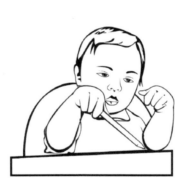

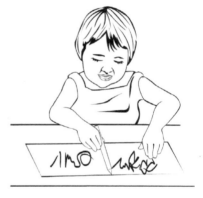

12 months: Imitative artist at work. Typical grasp of pencil at its proximal end with right hand with 'mirror' posturing in left hand. A moment later the pencil was passed from right to left, again marking paper.

15 months: Firmer grasp of the pencil now and held lower down the shaft, end product of to and fro lines and dots is improved. Mirror posture in left hand.

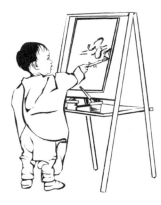

21 months: Larger brushwork at an easel. Productions are still more in the nature of visuo-motor activities than representative pictures.

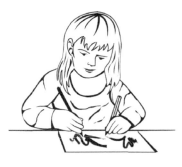

3½ years: Interesting example of simultaneous two-handed performance. The pencil grip near tip is more mature, but the production is still non-pictorial.

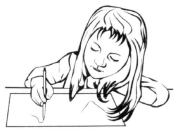

3½ years: Right-handed mature grip of pencil with non-engagement of left. The child asked to be given a letter to copy. They did not seem to realize that what had been copied was upside down.

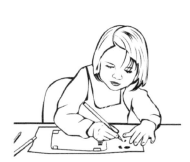

4 years: Drawing a typical age-characteristic house with cornered windows, simultaneously thinking aloud about it. The mature grip of right hand and the helpful use of left (to steady the paper) are well shown.

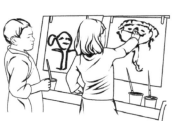

3½ and 4 years: Painting human figures. One used only black paint, the other several colours. The end products are both fairly age-characteristic. Originally reported these as self-portraits, but cheerfully admitted many inaccuracies.

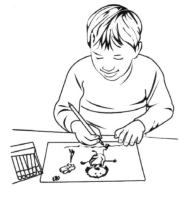

4¾ years: The child produces a colourful self-portrait with numerous common environmental embellishments – yellow sun, blue sky, green trees, brown earth. They print their name beneath, working briskly and silently in happy concentration.

**Summary -
mark making**

Of note in the sequence of mark making activity from 12 months to three years is the development of fine motor control and the exploration of the mark making object with both hands. We can see how fine motor control develops as the child tentatively holds the tip of the pencil through to their later adopting a competent grasp, further down the shaft. Despite hand preference normally being apparent at around 2 years of age or before (Michel *et al.*, 2016), in the case of these mark making examples, children seem to experiment with both hands through mirrored action. For example, in the first two drawings, the children explore the mark making object and in the fourth image, the child makes marks simultaneously with both hands. The emphasis at this early stage is on the process of mark making rather than on the production of anything representative. As children begin to become interested in drawing particular things, their hand preference becomes more apparent, seemingly as the increased control allows them to draw with increased precision. Children's first drawings are often of people and are relatively uniform in their presentation, comprising a circular body with facial features, and arms and legs stemming off. These are often termed tadpole figures or cephalopods (Cox, 2013). Interestingly however, these early drawings are not representative of young children's knowledge and understanding but rather, are schematic representations designed to communicate meaning. For example, just as in Sheridan's observation here, children often draw houses with a triangular roof, four-cornered windows (often with curtains) and a central door. This is despite not necessarily living or even seeing a house of this type.

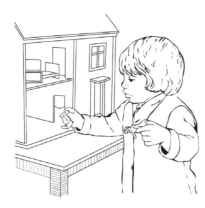

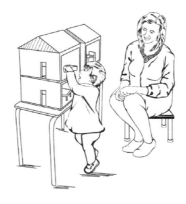

15 months: Miniature toys are merely small items to be manipulated and put in and out of an upright box-like container.

18 months: The miniature toys are objects for give-and-take play with the caregiver. The caregiver names toys and the child repeats the name but still does not appreciate that the toys represent real-life objects.

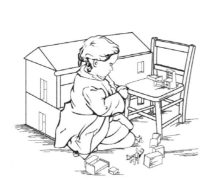

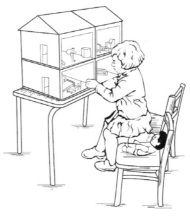

2½ years: The child knows that the toys are representative but prefers to assemble them in smaller, separated groups outside the dolls' house.

3¼ years: The child plays with the miniatures inside one room of the house, carrying on a long, audible monologue for their own and their doll's benefit.

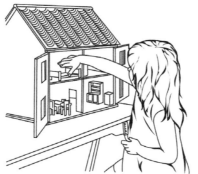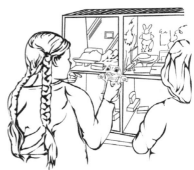

5 years: Playing constructively all over the house. Although silent, they are busily engaged.

6 and 6½ years: 'Special friends', they said, engaged in elaborate, co-operative, make-believe play in the dolls' house. The play goes on continuously from day to day. They had papered the walls and made all of the furnishings themselves.

Summary – small world play

In this final sequence of observations, Sheridan focuses on children's use of small objects associated with pretend play. There is some evidence to suggest that pretend play helps to support the development of language skills, socialization and emotional wellbeing (Lillard *et al.*, 2013). At 15 months, the child plays with the objects indiscriminately, merely placing them in and out of the house just as they would with other small items and a container. This type of placing and sorting is common in early childhood and is often repetitious. Later, with the presence of an adult, there appears to be evidence of the play cycle (Sturrock & Else, 1998), where the child and adult take turns to pass the objects to one another. Here, there is also imitation of object naming. Being able to attach labels to the objects, at two and a half, the child now appreciates that they are representative of real life objects. Piaget proposed that changes in cognition and understanding facilitated the development of language skill. In contrast, Vygotsky (1978) suggested the reverse, that language development supported thinking skills. For Vygotsky, children first externalize their thought processes by talking through their actions. Then, over time, internal speech is used to guide behaviour. This shift can be seen in Sheridan's fourth and fifth observations. At three and a half, despite being alone, the child pursues a long dialogue as they play. At age five however, whilst still alone, they are deeply engaged but remain silent. In the final observation, we see evidence of older children's progression from solitary to co-operative play (Parten, 1932).

■ Spend some time observing children of different ages engaged with the same play materials.

- How does their play differ?

- What do they play?

- How long do they play for?

- Who do they play with?

- How do they use the materials?

■ What different skills and abilities do the children of different ages show in relation to the main areas of development? Think about:

- Social and emotional skills

- Language and communication

- Cognitive development

- Fine and gross motor skill

Give yourself some time to think

5   Variation in children's play

Consistent with Sheridan's original focus, this chapter will consider play and atypical development. It will present some examples of atypical development, how these may impact on children's play and the way in which play could be tailored to suit individual needs. In addition, it will include a discussion of variation in play according to gender, culture and adversity.

The specific aims of the chapter are:

- To highlight some of the key issues relating to play according to gender, culture, atypical development and adversity.

- To consider the value of understanding variation apparent in play in relation to professional play practice and providing for play.

Culture

Understanding variation in play is important because it provides an insight into the uniqueness of different cultures, facilitates culturally appropriate professional practice, and highlights the dynamic and ever-changing structure and social organization of families (Roopnarine *et al.*, 1998). Through her observations, Sheridan demonstrates how children develop a repertoire of play behaviours, this repertoire growing with children's increasing social, physical, intellectual and emotional competencies. Children across all cultures play in the ways described by Sheridan, developing a repertoire of skills to support play that involves the use of senses, objects, symbolism and pretence, and an understanding of rules. Sheridan's original observations of the universal play types children engage in are consistent with current reviews of children's play behaviour as discussed in chapter 1 (e.g. Whitebread, 2012). As Hughes (2010) states, play is a true cultural universal and even children with substantial domestic or agricultural duties seem to find opportunities to play during their day (Maybin & Woodhead, 2003). An anthropological study by Watson-Gegeo (2001) illustrates how children in Kwara-ae appear to switch from 'child mode' to 'adult mode' throughout their day, in order to make time to both play and complete their work duties. However, although there appears no cultural variation in the development of children's *ability to play*, culture both influences and is manifested in children's *play behaviour*. Variation that exists in children's play behaviour both within and across cultures is likely to reflect the way adults interact with their children, with differing emphasis placed on the value and function of play and provision for play.

As has been previously noted, parents or primary caregivers often serve as a baby's first playmate. The literature surrounding parenting behaviour suggests that cultural variations exist in the nature of early interactions between children and their primary caregivers (Roopnarine, 2012; Webb, 2013). Of importance to the process of developing play skills, however, is that effective early parent-child interactions serve to ensure that the child feels emotionally secure and able to explore their social and material environment (Jennings, 2011). Lieberman (1977) talked of parents and teachers as 'cultural surrogates', inhibiting or encouraging children's play. In a review of the literature on parent-child interaction during play, O'Reilly and Bornstein (1993) demonstrated that the level of sophistication in children's play was related to the quality and nature of early parent-child interactions. Further, Milteer *et al.* (2012) make a compelling case for the importance of play for developing secure attachment bonds. Effective early interactions are characterized by the provision of boundaries and emotional responsiveness. Roopnarine (2012) and Webb (2013) remind us that parenting occurs within a cultural context, and the way that parents express emotional responsiveness and set boundaries in play often reflects parenting practice which itself is deeply embedded within a cultural context. Hughes (2010) describes how American mothers tend to set broad boundaries in play, encouraging children to take notice of and explore the wider environment, consistent with their promotion of autonomy and independence. By contrast, he describes how Japanese mothers tend to encourage play that involves close and controlled social interaction, such as nurturing doll play, promoting a sense of dependency.

Haight *et al.* (1999) also describe how the themes of pretend play reflect socialization goals: for example, European and American caregivers emphasize individuality, self-expression and independence, while Chinese caregivers emphasize harmonious social interaction, obedience, respect and rules. The transmission of cultural values through play is evident in the specific content of children's pretend play behaviour. Gosso (2010) for example, discusses how the pretend play of children from hunter-gatherer communities in Brazil, tends to focus on the imitation of adult activities. This provides an example of how cultural values are transmitted through play, facilitating children's sense of belonging and citizenship.

Cultural variation is also evident in the emphasis placed on play within education. In China, play was historically seen as recreational rather than educational and not related to intellectual development (Cooney & Sha, 1999). Whereas messy play areas are common to early years classrooms in the United Kingdom, David and Powell (2005) found that Chinese practitioners failed to understand why an area that encouraged children to get dirty should be promoted as it contradicted the principles of cleanliness and order. More recent research however, suggests that there is now increasing recognition that play serves a useful developmental function in terms of social skills (Li *et al.,* 2016) and physical development (Hua *et al.*, 2016). It also has a more prominent role in early years provision, with Chinese teachers being actively engaged in planning and supporting children's play (Yang, 2013).

Variation also exists in the availability or suitability of play materials. Lindon (2001) describes how, in some cultures, dolls hold particular spiritual or ceremonial significance and as such might not be considered suitable for play. Where toys are not available for play, children will often construct what they need from materials found in their environment. Play materials in Kenya among Massai children, for example, include toys made from wood, straw, animal skins and bone, stones, and other found objects. Sometimes props are not needed at all and play revolves solely around shared knowledge and understanding (Haight *et al.*, 1999): for example, in the development of game-playing rules in street culture (Sobel, 2001; Fearn & Howard, 2011). At the other end of the spectrum,

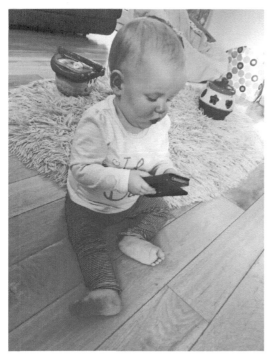

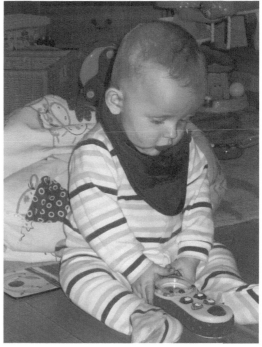

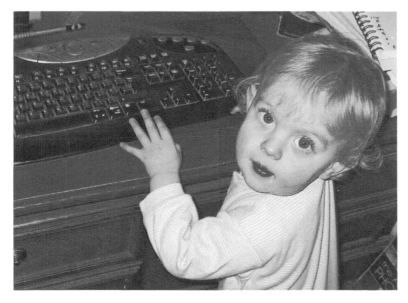

Even at a young age, these children know how the electronic devices at home are used. Toy versions of computers and mobile phones allow them to incorporate real life into their play.

the influence of our technological world is reflected in the replica toys made available for even the youngest children: for example, pretend mobile phones and baby laptops. The miniaturization of the technology associated with consumer electronics means that children may now interact with sophisticated materials as they play.

There is a growing body of research into both the negative and positive consequences of technological play (e.g. Howard-Jones, 2011). Research has demonstrated that the quality of mother-child interactions can be reduced when play involves technological toys (Wooldridge & Shapka, 2012). When balanced with other more traditional types of play and carefully monitored and managed by parents however, Plowman and McPake (2013) highlight how digital play has the potential to contribute to children's development in multiple ways.

Globalization and an increasingly multicultural society are also reflected in children's play. The festivities associated with Halloween, a celebration that involves dressing up as ghosts and ghouls and playing such games as apple-bobbing and trick or treat, originated in American culture but have since spread to many other parts of the world. Play in an East Indian context is often influenced by ceremonial activities, such as the celebration of Diwali, where children and families tell ancient stories through puppetry, music and dance, and celebrate colour and light through mark making and fireworks (Roopnarine *et al.*, 1998). In a growing multicultural society, these celebrations are increasingly likely to be shared by children and families from a variety of backgrounds, through community activities and school experiences.

Gender influences and is manifested in children's play behaviour in much the same way as culture. Variation reflects adult interactions with children, children's interactions with each other as well as gendered norms and values projected through marketing and the media.

Gender

The words 'gender' and 'sex' are often used interchangeably. For example, on forms or questionnaires we may be asked to tick a box to indicate our 'gender' as being male or female. The response required, however, relates to our biological sex. Arguably, gender relates to the characteristics associated with our biological sex, characteristics which are often learned via the process of socialization. Distinguishing between sex and gender in research is important as findings relating to sex differences would suggest variation between boys and girls from a biological or genetic perspective, whereas findings relating to gender difference would include variation resulting from the process of socialization. As the development of play skills is largely a social process, unpicking that which is a result of biological sex and that which is a result of socialization can be difficult, if not impossible. If we consider the observations of Sheridan in relation to the social, physical, intellectual and linguistic competencies associated with the developing repertoire of play skills, then, from a biological perspective, boys and girls progress in much the same way. Variation is more apparent in relation to what they choose to play.

Research has consistently demonstrated that, given a choice of toys to play with, children show a preference for those that are commonly associated with their own gender (Weisgram *et al.*, 2014). Servin *et al.* (1999) demonstrated that these gendered choices became apparent as early as 12 months. However, even at this young age, it is still difficult to conclude that the behaviour is a result of any differences due to biological sex. Returning to Sheridan's point about parents acting as children's first play partners, it seems likely that, in a more general sense, styles of interaction with children from birth could contribute to the development of their gendered toy preferences. Mothers and fathers have been shown to interact with their children in subtly different ways, with mothers tending towards intimate communicative forms of interaction and fathers tending towards more physical activity (John *et al.*, 2013). The gender of the child also influences the style of our interactions. Lindahl and Heimann (1997) studied the social behaviour of mother-daughter and mother-son dyads and found that mother-daughter dyads remained in closer proximity to one another and engaged in more physical and visual contact. It may be that the close proximity and intimate communication apparent in interaction with baby girls lends itself to nurturing types of play while the emphasis on physical activity and opportunities for independence and exploration are reflected in boys choosing to play with mobile toys, such as cars and trucks.

Interestingly, gendered differences in day-to-day parent-child interactions reduce with age, perhaps because they have served their purpose in provoking children's initial awareness of being male or female. However, Lindsey *et al.* (2010) found that, despite showing no gender differences in day-to-day caregiver interaction, parents continued to engage in gendered patterns of behaviour with their children during play. Rogoff (2003) explains that young children actively develop their understanding of gender through play, exploring the concepts of 'boy' and 'girl' and acting out the extremes of each role. As well as imitating what they see in their home environments, a widened social network coupled with exposure to television broadcasting reinforces their gender knowledge. Differences are manifest within more complex types of play, for example in the types of role-playing games in which they choose to engage and in the specific roles they adopt within this play.

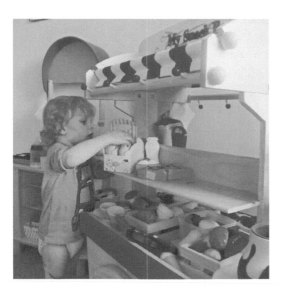

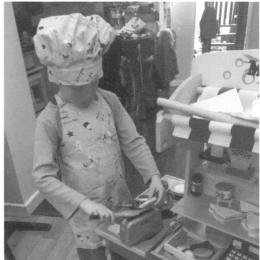

At age 2, this young boy enjoyed sorting and stacking the play materials on the shopping cart.

Later, at age 4, he fully engaged in pretend play, preparing a meal. Whilst shopping and cooking may once have been considered female gendered play, in contemporary society this is far less likely.

The patterns of preferential toy choice made in the first year extend into later childhood, where girls seek out information about human relationships and boys seek out action (Kalliala, 2006). Research has demonstrated that gendered behaviour becomes increasingly rigid at around 3–4 years of age in terms of toy choice and the themes that are enacted during pretend play (Halim *et al.*, 2013). Boys' tendency to engage in more rough-and-tumble activity is perhaps the most widely documented gender variation in children's play. Research has consistently shown that across cultures, boys tend to engage in more of this physical type of play than girls (Jarvis, 2006). Themes in role play among boys also tend to involve war or pseudo-violence, and much has been done in the United Kingdom to curtail this type of activity. However, there is no clear evidence that engagement in this type of play leads to future violence (Holland, 2003) and, as we saw in the previous section, children are likely to follow their desired play patterns even in the absence of props, either doing without or making toys out of found items.

Adversity and atypicality

It seems unlikely that variation in the spontaneous development of children's play behaviour is directly influenced by gender or culture. While the content of their play may differ, boys and girls across all cultures develop the physical, cognitive, social and linguistic capacities to play in the variety of ways described by Sheridan. Any differences in the predominance of play behaviour according to gender or culture, in the main, appear to emerge as a result of environmental stimuli and the assimilation of cultural norms and values: for example, through the availability of materials, parenting behaviour, peer interaction or exposure to the media. Observations of children's play among those facing severe adversity or those who have particular developmental needs may be more likely to indicate different or disrupted patterns of play behaviour.

Sheridan describes how, with adequate opportunity and support, children gain mastery over their actions, integrating sensory and motor experiences. This mastery builds esteem and confidence, and children spontaneously seek out new challenges. They use their existing play skills and emotional security as resources to support future development. Although not necessarily the case, adversity and atypicality can alter or interrupt this process.

In the case of adversity, children may not be provided with the opportunity to play or to create a strong emotional base through secure attachments. Webb and Brown (2003) demonstrated how regular interaction with others and being offered opportunities to play greatly improved the development of children who had previously been confined to hospital beds in Romania. Alternatively, children may face such severe disruption that the prospect of a new challenge overwhelms them and they may stop playing or return to early play behaviours with which they feel comfortable. According to Hyder (2005), the majority of children can be helped to overcome adversity through their own play. After the 2006 Lebanese war, UNICEF funded the development of recreational areas to restore children's play behaviours and found that reintroducing opportunities to play in a safe space contributed greatly to children's wellbeing. In a series of cross-cultural case studies, Fearn and Howard (2012) describe how during periods of stress, children actively sought out play opportunities, building resilience to overcome the challenges of their daily lives. Following the Christchurch earthquakes, Bateman, Danby and Howard (2013) identified how children's wellbeing was supported by them playing out their traumatic experiences. Of course, for some children, specialist support is necessary and complex trauma might involve children working with play therapists or psychotherapists. Here, play is employed more directly as a means of communicating and resolving emotional issues.

Atypically developing children may have physical disabilities, sensory, social or intellectual impairment or a combination of these things, which makes integrating learning experiences more challenging. Writing about deaf children, Marschark (1993) suggests that in a bid to view disability more positively, we can often dismiss what he terms self-evident truths, in that atypically developing children often experience a more limited world, their interactions are guided by different rules and constraints and these differences are likely to impact on their development in complex and numerous ways. He proposes that the key issue is to look beyond superficial differences to those that have functional significance, those that impact on children's development and subsequent life experiences. From a developmental perspective, children with sensory, social and intellectual impairments often show a preference for more solitary or parallel types of play and engage in less imaginative role play or symbolic play with objects (Howard & McInnes, 2013a). More important than observing differences in children's play patterns, however, is understanding why these differences occur, whether these differences are likely to impact on achievement, enjoyment and quality of life and, if so, whether support based on children's abilities can be tailored to broaden skills and experiences. Unpacking the social, cognitive, linguistic and physical demands of play and reflecting on children's potential to meet these demands mean we are better able to provide play opportunities that are appropriately challenging but do not risk frustration, boredom or emotional distress. In addition, as was highlighted in chapter 1, it is useful to remember the complexities that surround what does or does not, constitute play behaviour. Whilst not fitting traditional play typologies, Eisele and Howard (2012) identified many play like cues in the ritual repetitive behaviour of children with autism. Table 1 highlights the way that certain developmental difficulties or disabilities might impact on play, and gives some ideas of how we might tailor play experiences to best meet these children's needs. There is not scope to consider every type of challenge a child might face in an introductory text such as this, and it goes without saying that an individual case-by-case approach is required in order to provide the best care and support possible.

Children can be helped to overcome adversity and to make the most of their play with considered support that builds on their strengths and abilities. Considered support will undoubtedly involve parents and professionals working with children in partnership, providing for enjoyment of the here and now of play, as well as supporting developmental progress. Sheridan remarks that 'some of the so-called play pressed upon atypically developing children, always with the best intention, has been perilously close to drudgery' (1977, p. 13). It is important that we do not overemphasize play as a way of becoming, at the detriment to play as a way of being (Howard & McInnes, 2013a). We must remain mindful that a sense of freedom, choice and control is paramount to the broad range of play experiences we offer to all children (Howard, 2010b).

Table 5.1 Characteristics of some types of developmental challenge and their implications for play activity

Developmental Challenge	Potential characteristics	Implications relating to play	Examples of play activities
ADHD	Poor attention, hyperactivity or impulsive behaviour	Delayed play skills, shorter episodes of sustained play, difficulties with social relationships and accepting rules, increased risky activity	Play in open spaces to expend energy, gradually increase turn taking and interaction, extend self chosen play activities, offer limited choice to avoid overstimulation
ASD	Difficulties with social relationships and communication skills, the presence of ritual-repetitive behaviour	Preference for solitary activity, routine and familiarity, lower level of imaginative or pretend play, discomfort with sensory activity	Talk to the child about their play, use familiar activities (including ritual repetitive behaviour) as the starting point for co-operative play, gradually introduce sensory experiences
Down Syndrome	General developmental delay across domains particularly fine and gross motor skills, the potential for heart, vision and hearing difficulties	Delayed development of play skills, preference for familiar activities, difficulties with co-ordination and manipulating play materials	Use self chosen play activities as a starting point for introducing new materials, encourage play that supports the development of gross and fine motor skills
Vision / hearing / speech impairment	Full or partially blind or deaf, difficulties with speech production, stutter, language delay	More time needed to make sense of the environment, preference for solitary activity, communication difficulties, less imaginative play	Introduce a variety of sensory activities, encourage turn taking and interaction, in the case of speech issues, model language rich play
Developmental disorders that present physical challenges	Specific to particular conditions but, for example, co-ordination and muscle control difficulties, issues relating to respiratory or digestive functioning, increased susceptibility to common childhood illnesses	Mobility difficulties, frequent hospitalization, under developed play skills, low levels of confidence and independence	Provide activities that enable children to make choices to develop autonomy and self esteem, encourage the manipulation of materials that demonstrate cause and effect, provide play opportunities that support physical development and co-ordination

Adapted from Howard & McInnes, (2013a) The Essence of Play: A Practice Companion for Professionals Working with Children and Young People

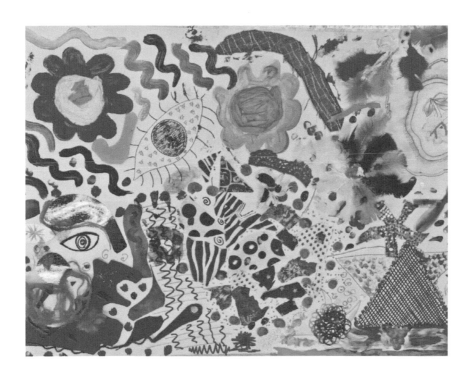

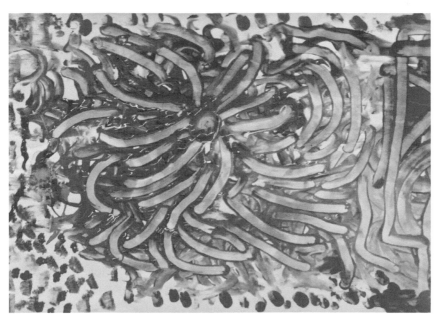

Art and craft can be a useful medium for children to express their emotions and work through challenging experiences.

Inclusive play practice

Sheridan's observations of real children engaged in their own spontaneous play reveal how social, physical, linguistic and cognitive competencies gradually accrue, to enable increasingly complex forms of play. Development of and through play reflects the increasingly effective integration of sensory and motor experiences, and these experiences are supported by social interaction. Information based on developmental milestones often feeds into targets for attainment, and it has been argued that this emphasizes a top-down or deficit model of development that focuses on the skills children have yet to achieve, rather than their current abilities (Lindon, 2001). However, understanding the skills associated with children's behaviour is important even in a bottom-up approach. At a basic level it allows us to plan the experiences and materials we might make available for children; but, importantly, it also helps us to understand and support their development better. Young children's development is best supported through play as it enables children to explore the world around them and offers rich opportunities for social interaction. However, enabling children to learn through play relies on our understanding that play itself is a developmental process and, like other developmental processes, is subject to variation. Play behaviours and play skills can be indicative of and/or influenced by culture, atypicality and adversity. Best practice recognizes children's growing *ability to play* as well as supporting their *development through play*.

Throughout this book we have been reminded that while children learn in lots of different ways, the sense of freedom, choice and control inherent in play renders it particularly useful for development. When children are at play, their development is enhanced. Remaining mindful of these characteristics can ensure inclusive and supportive play practice. Most notably, good practice starts with the child and emphasizes achievement rather than attainment (DfES, 2001; APPG, 2015). If we seek to promote activities that afford a sense of freedom, choice and control, we can be more certain that our practice begins with the child. We can support children's application of what they know and can do, fostering their personal learning journeys. Inclusive play practice is accessible to all children and allows them to demonstrate achievement, whatever their ability. As will be discussed in the following chapter, adults have an important role in supporting children's play experiences. They make decisions as to the time, space and materials made available for safe play, accommodating and supporting children's repertoire of play skills. They recognize the value of children's own initiated activities and understand factors that might influence or be manifested in children's play. They negotiate their position as a play partner, responding sensitively to children's play cues to maintain or extend the play flow. Supporting children's *ability to play*, as well as promoting their *development through play*, involves constant reflection.

Establishing a partnership with the child and their family ensures that we begin planning play experiences with as much knowledge as possible. Information can be shared across multidisciplinary teams and might consider:

■ cultural values and beliefs;

■ family structure;

■ strengths and challenges: social, physical, cognitive, linguistic and emotional;

■ likes and dislikes;

■ any issues of adversity.

Information gained from talking to the child, their parents or other professionals is combined with expertise in child development and play, to guide planning and provision. This might consider:

■ What kinds of experiences will best support the child? Why?

■ What kinds of activities and materials are suitable? Why?

■ Do planned experiences support ability to play as well as development through play?

■ Do the experiences afford the child a sense of freedom, choice and control?

■ What will your role be in these activities and how will this be managed?

Once play is ongoing, a constant process of reflection informs developmental progress, future planning and our own professional development. This might include planned, opportunistic, structured or unstructured observations and talking to children about their play, perhaps using photographs or artefacts as conversational prompts. It might involve thinking about time, space and materials for play or about our own role in play activities. Some questions to ask might include:

■ How enjoyable or desirable are the activities?

■ How are spaces and materials being used?

■ Is the child able to employ current skills? Can they develop new ones?

■ How do the observations feed into knowledge of the child in relation to previously noted strengths and weaknesses?

■ What was your role in the play? Was this as planned? Was it effective?

Summary

■ All children seem to engage in play.

■ Play reflects cultural norms and values.

■ Socialization can influence children's play preferences.

■ Play can help children to overcome adversity.

■ Inclusive play practice fosters ability to play as well as development through play.

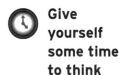

Give yourself some time to think

■ Take some time to research a culture that is different to your own.

   – Do you find anything that might impact on children's play or your own play practice?

■ Next time you are watching television or reading a magazine, look out for gendered information.

   – Towards whom is the material directed? What impact might this have on children's developing gender identity?

- Research one type of developmental difficulty or disability.

- How might this impact on the child's development?

- In what ways could play experiences be tailored to suit the child's needs?

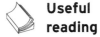
Useful reading

Hyder, T. (2005). *War, conflict and play*. Maidenhead: Open University Press.

Macintyre, C. (2009). *Play for children with special needs: Supporting children with learning differences*. Sussex: Routledge.

Roopnarine *et al.* (eds). (2014). *International perspectives on children's play*. Maidenhead: Open University Press.

6   Providing for play

This chapter will focus on the ways in which children's development can be supported through play. Extending our discussion of reflective practice from the previous chapter, we will consider the importance of play for the development of secure attachment bonds and the different roles adults might adopt when playing with children. We will consider the value and importance of play across a variety of contexts that might be encountered by children as they grow. In addition, we will explore the work of play professionals within these contexts.

The specific aims of the chapter are:

■ To highlight the importance of play for the development of healthy attachment bonds.

  – To consider provision for play in relation to adult roles, opportunities for social interaction and available resources such as space, time and play materials.

■ To explore the roles of different play professions and the theoretical underpinnings of these roles.

Provisions for play

Sheridan (1977) identifies four provisions as being of primary importance to enable spontaneous play: playthings, playspace, playtime and playmates.

> Sheridan (1977) writes:
>
> ■ *Playthings* must be appropriate for the child's age and stage of growth and development. Not too few or the child will lack stimulation, and not too many or they will become confused and unable to concentrate.

- *Playspace* is needed for the 'free-ranging' activities which are commonly shared with others, but every child must also possess a small personal 'territory' which they know is their own and provides a secure home base.

- *Playtime* must be reasonably peaceful and predictable. It should be adequate for fulfillment of whatever activity is engaging the child's interest, without premature interruption likely to cause frustration, or undue prolongation leading to boredom, loneliness or feeling of neglect.

- *Playfellows* are required at all stages of development. Encouraging adults are not only essential to dependent infants but also in the period of *solo-play* which is characteristic of children under 2½ years, who are still unaware of such abstract principles as equal rights, sharing and taking turns. The need for companionship proceeds as social communications improve.

Playthings

In commercial society, we can often feel overwhelmed with toys designed to have pre-planned outcomes that promote cultural materialistic values. Items with such fixed purposes often appear to contradict the notion of spontaneity in play. Indeed, sometimes these items place a strong emphasis on developmental or educational outcomes rather than offering real play value. Hyun (1998) suggests that parents from European and North American backgrounds often value play for its potential to promote cognitive development and that this influences them when choosing toys for their children. Boekee and Brown (2015) also found that choice of toys, particularly in relation to their being gender specific, differs according to whether or not the adult is a parent. However, in chapter 1, we saw how the same activity could be seen as play or not play by children, where the approach taken to the activity is more important than the materials themselves. Children's playthings are often the simplest of items, objects that can be used flexibly in a variety of ways. Fabrics of different colours and textures stimulate the senses and at the same time provide endless ideas for dressing up. As Sheridan demonstrates in her observations, cardboard boxes can be climbed into and out of as children learn about their relative size, and they can be used to make dens or other constructions. Den building has been shown to be favourite play activity for children across time and culture (Kamp, 2015) and provides children with rich opportunities for developing creative problem solving skills and imagination (Canning, 2013).

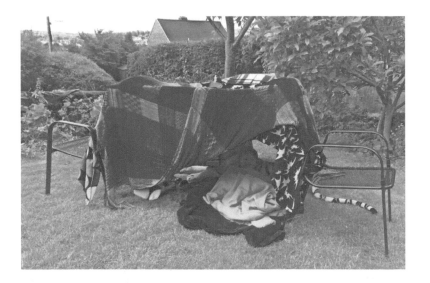

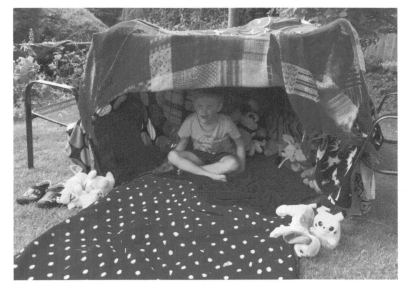

This 6-year-old enjoyed making a den with chairs, pegs and blankets. What started as quite a basic structure soon transformed into a very comfortable space to sit and play!

Children can make great use of household items and will often choose these over plastic imitations, preferring real saucepans and spoons in their imitative domestic play. Saucepans and spoons are also ideal for noise making. Random collections of items in a box or basket *invite* rather than *direct* the young child to explore objects and their properties (Goldschmied & Jackson, 1994; Gascoyne, 2012).

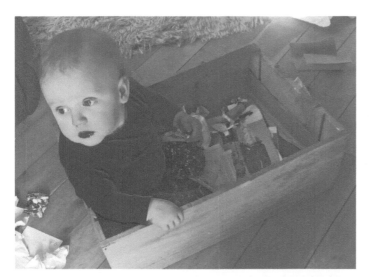

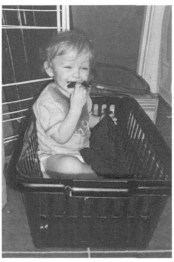

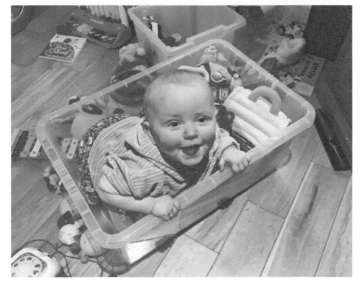

Children enjoy climbing into boxes of all kinds, learning about their relative size.

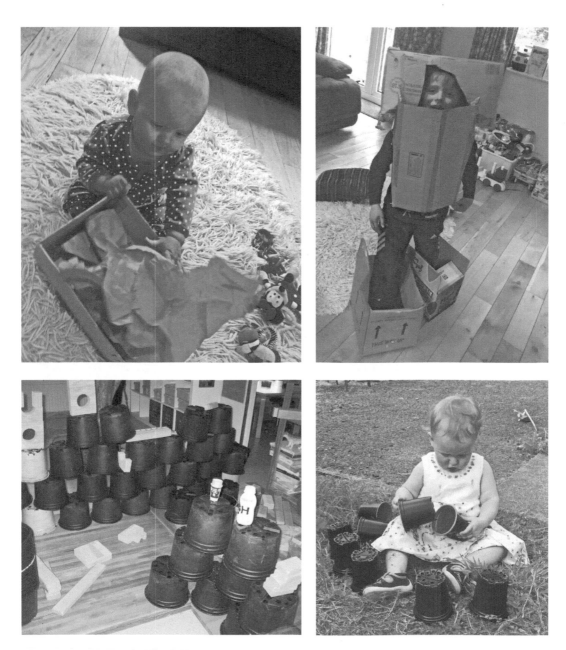

Playthings need not be expensive or complex. Children can make great use of 'loose parts' such as scraps of material, cardboard boxes or old plant pots.

Children being creative with items that are not restricted by a particular use is framed within Nicholson's theory of loose parts (1971). This emphasizes the value of offering children open-ended and often natural play materials that give them the opportunity to develop their play – introducing, modifying and changing ideas. This is an idea that has been long been incorporated into open access playwork settings and adventure playgrounds, but can now also be frequently observed in nursery and school playgrounds. Research demonstrates that offering 'loose parts' such as cardboard boxes, fabrics, wooden planks or crates can have beneficial effects, for example reducing sedentary activity during playtimes (Engelen *et al.*, 2013) and increasing collaboration, creativity and concentration when back in class (Yavuz, 2016).

When choosing materials for play, it is useful to consider their purpose and play value and their potential for open and closed use. Of course, materials must always be safe for children and checked frequently for wear and tear.

Time and space

When creating time and space for play, it is useful to be aware that children become attuned to details such as where, when and with whom activities take place, and they learn to distinguish play from other activities through their experiences (Howard & McInnes, 2013a). To encourage children to take a playful approach to a wide range of activities, adults can ensure that play is not restricted to a particular location, unnecessarily timed, socially prescriptive or secondary to other activities. Time available for play need not be excessive and children seek out opportunities to play amid the busiest of schedules. If children are in control of their play, the potential for them to become bored, restless or prematurely interrupted is kept to a minimum.

Sheridan stresses the importance of both shared and personal spaces for children's play. Children need space where they can play with others but also smaller, quiet spaces for their own solitary activity, providing opportunities for autonomy and independence but also a secure base to which they can return or retreat, as and when necessary. Indoor and outdoor places are both important. Children seek adventure and challenge in their play outdoors; they explore places and enjoy transforming spaces to create imaginary worlds (Tovey,

2007; Wilson, 2012). A particular challenge is providing play spaces that stimulate children's abilities within the boundaries of health, safety and wellbeing (Brussoni *et al.*, 2012).

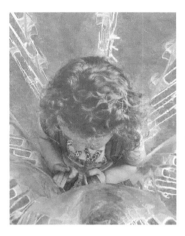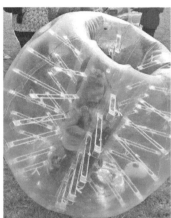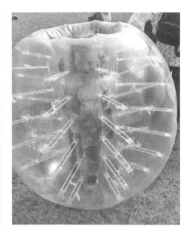

In a large outdoor space, being in a 'zorb ball' gave this 4-year-old a challenging new physical experience.

Partners in play

Living and learning with others are essential skills for life. As is documented in chapter 1, play becomes increasingly social over time. Interacting with others in play increases children's social skills, an awareness of self and an awareness of cultural norms and values.

Parents/carers and siblings

A newborn baby is able to communicate and respond to their mother's voice, face, touch, taste and smell. Mothers appear inherently prepared to respond to their babies, form a lasting attachment, and are sensitive to their babies' needs. Spontaneous play often involves primary carers being the baby's best toy. Some scholars even argue that the development of attachment bonds through the playful interaction between a mother and child begins in utero, and has a powerful effect on the developing brain (Jennings, 2011). Early interactions encourage social interaction and playfulness, for example peek-a-boo and imitation games soon become the source of much fun and amusement for young infants. These playful interactions are particularly important for the development of attachments, which enable the young child to feel secure enough to explore the world around them (Milteer *et al.*, 2012).

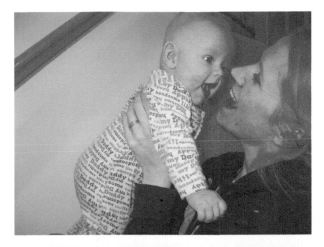

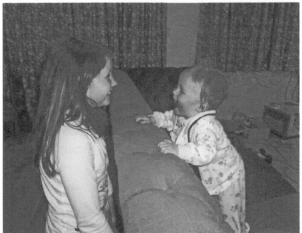

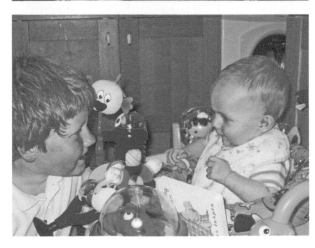

Early interactions between babies and their parents/carers and siblings are important. Healthy attachment bonds provide a sense of security for children to explore the world around them.

Quality parent-child interaction involves listening to, respecting and supporting the child to encourage an exploration of strengths and limitations within secure boundaries. The importance of secure attachment bonds is such that there has been a significant growth in programmes designed to facilitate the development of close parent-child relationships. Examples include baby massage classes, language and play sessions, music and rhyme groups or classes based on sensory activities. All of these encourage parents or carers to interact with their babies in playful ways, recognizing and responding to cues so as to nurture opportunities for bonding.

Peers and friendships

Friendship longevity develops over time. Young children often refer to playmates as their friends. For example, when a 3-year-old says, 'I am your friend now', it probably means 'I am playing with you now' (Dowling, 2000). Children develop a closeness to friends interested in playing the same games through shared play experiences. Initial friendship choices are based on proximity and being playmates. During this play, however, children develop the skills necessary to learn about themselves and others, enabling them to make friendship decisions based on personal characteristics. Recent research suggests that peers become a particularly important determinant of how playful activities are in middle childhood (Howard *et al.*, 2017). Whilst traditionally, definitions of play have suggested activities must be freely chosen, further research suggests that in reality, the choice about what, with whom, where or when to play is often negotiated with peers (King & Howard, 2014), demonstrating the importance of play for the development of life long social skills.

Other adults

Lindon (2001) identifies the important roles adopted by adults in play, including:

■ Play partner – becoming an equal in the play

■ Observer – observing children's development and progress

■ Admirer – showing that you value the play

■ Facilitator – easing play along

- Model – showing how play materials might be used

- Mediator – resolving conflict

- Safety officer – ensuring safety

Taking on a range of roles is important. A predominantly mediating or modelling role can influence whether children accept adults into their play on future occasions (Howard, 2002; Howard & McInnes, 2013a). Engaging as an equal partner in play affords children an authentic sense of control and communicates that we value their own self-initiated activities. The nature of the dialogue that occurs is also important. Particular types of question posing can enable possibility thinking and creativity (Chappell *et al.*, 2008) and teachers who use open-ended questions and authentic dialogue are more likely to be accepted by children as play partners (McInnes *et al.*, 2013)

Large-scale research has demonstrated the importance of high-quality adult-child interactions in early years settings for children's development (Sylva *et al.*, 2010). Stepping back and listening to the child offers empowerment; the child is in a position to take control in decision-making, rather than following the adult's lead. Being sensitive, showing respect and taking an empathetic stance will allow the practitioner and child to establish a trusting relationship. The child will feel sufficiently safe to take risks that are framed by a shared understanding of boundaries. Here it is useful to return to the notion of the play cycle introduced in chapter 1. To facilitate prolonged and rich child-directed play experiences, adults must identify and respond appropriately to, the child's play cues, maximizing opportunities for development across domains.

Play in different contexts

The opportunities for development within authentic play activities cannot be neatly compartmentalized. Play supports children's development across multiple domains.

Sheridan (1977) writes:

Play provides opportunities to strengthen the body, improve the mind, develop the personality and acquire social competence, it is as necessary as food, warmth and protective care. It represents:

- *Apprenticeship*, i.e. practice leading to competence in everyday skills.

- *Research*, i.e. observation, exploration, speculation and discovery.

- *Occupational therapy*, i.e. relief from pain, boredom or distress.

- *Recreation*, i.e. simple, enjoyable fun.

Opportunities for apprenticeship, research, occupational therapy and recreation exist in all play, particularly when children are afforded freedom, choice and control. However, various play professionals emphasize opportunities differently. For example, the educational value of play has traditionally focused far more on the role of play for exploration, discovery and the development of skills, features of Sheridan's apprenticeship and research roles.

Educational play   One of the first advocates of play in early education was Froebel (1782–1852). Froebel designed particular materials to support what he described as the occupation of play. As a result, his ideas are often interpreted as being structured and focused on skills development. This was certainly true for Montessori (1870–1952), who developed sets of apparatus to stimulate physical and sensory ability. Froebel, however, argued that play was the highest form of human expression and paid particular attention to the importance of open-ended play experiences for supporting personal and emotional development. Isaacs (1932) shared this view, and argued that the autonomy afforded to children in play supported a positive sense of self which, in turn, promoted intellectual development. Publishing in the same era, Piaget, who argued that play was secondary to real learning, became better known. He suggested that children's development could be documented in stages and that particular abilities and ways of thinking begin to emerge at key times. Of importance was that this pattern of development would unfold without the need for instruction and that children benefited from being active in their own learning. His focus on the nature of cognition, while invaluable for increasing knowledge of child development, translated into age-related practices and the need for activities to work towards promoting children's achievement of particular skills. His emphasis on the child's active role translated into discovery-based learning techniques but inadvertently led to a rather redundant role for practitioners.

Vygotsky (1978) placed stronger emphasis on the social and cultural elements of play. He suggested that play served as the first form of language and communication and that during play children learned to understand the nature of rules and symbols.

Social interaction was of particular importance and his notion of a zone of proximal development suggested that adults and more competent peers were able to support children's learning, enabling the completion of more complex tasks that they would eventually be able to complete alone. Although Vygotsky emphasized the social nature of learning, for him, children's own play activity served as a facilitator, much like the adult or more competent peer. Indeed, he argued that, in play, children behave as though they are a head taller than themselves.

The ideas of Piaget and Vygotsky are synthesized in the work of Bruner (1960). Heavily influenced by Piaget, Bruner proposed three different modes of exploration in early childhood:

- Enactive – direct manipulation of objects
- Iconic – mental manipulation of objects
- Symbolic – abstract manipulation of symbols

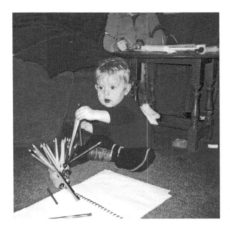 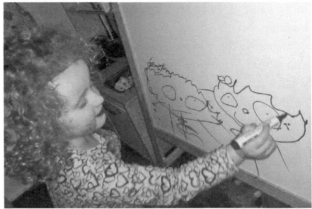

This infant imitates his sister, taking her pencils to make random marks on the paper. Later, at around three years, we can see how this little girl has learned to draw the human figure. These early tadpole like drawings are called cephalopods.

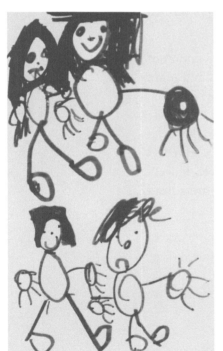 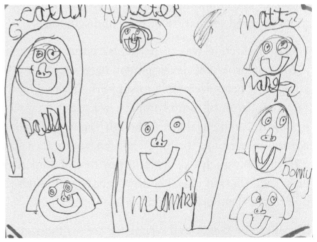

At around 4 years, these cephalopods become more complex before children develop their individual drawing style at around 6 years.

Mark making and drawing support the development of fine motor control skills and are one of the first ways children demonstrate symbolism. Mark making using a variety of different media is an important precursor to numeracy and literacy skills.

Bruner challenged the Piagetian idea that children needed to be ready for certain types of learning. He suggested that almost any concept could be introduced to children in some form at any time, and that the three different modes of exploration could be used without restriction. He argued that children needed to develop fundamental learning skills rather than facts, and that the best way to do this was via repeated exposure to basic ideas. In this spiral approach, children are able to extend their thinking, accruing skills and abilities that they can transfer to different contexts.

Within the realms of early education, play has been described as a principal vehicle for learning, and it is central to curriculum initiatives such as the Foundation Phase in Wales (DCELLS, 2008). Emphasis is placed on the development of the whole child, and teachers and classroom assistants must support children's development through the indoor and outdoor play opportunities they provide. Given the amount of time children spend in the school environment, teachers and classroom assistants are arguably our most important play professionals. Their jobs require extensive knowledge of play, learning and child development, and the skills to combine this successfully with the requirements of the curriculum.

Play professionals in education – Teachers, classroom assistants and therapeutic play specialists

Claire, nursery nurse, UK

I've been a nursery nurse for eleven years now and I started with a BTEC National Diploma qualification. I've seen many changes to the curriculum, and we are currently working with the Foundation Phase, which is a play-based approach. Balancing play provision with a need to show that children are learning can be hard work. We also have to balance the need for children to take risks with health and safety requirements, so many games and activities I remember playing are not allowed any more: conkers, marbles and climbing trees, for example. A particular challenge is making sure that staff are well trained. In education, the focus of training is often on learning and not much time is spent on play. I think good play practice relies on practitioners really understanding why play is important but there's not much training available. I've been proactive in developing my knowledge and have even started a higher degree in play. With my training and experience, I now value the process of play rather than focus on outcomes. I feel privileged when I am invited to join in children's activities, and I especially look forward to free play sessions. Of course, we do some structured activities too, but I try to make these playful by allowing children to take the lead. I feel more like an equal. There are often unexpected outcomes, and this is exciting.

There is also increasing recognition and research evidence to support the proposition that the freedom and choice inherent in play supports children's emotional and intellectual growth (Laevers, 1994; Howard & McInnes, 2013b). In primary school classrooms it is now increasingly common to see groups of children attending play based nurture groups or emotional development classes. For example, the Social and Emotional Aspects of Learning (SEAL) programme comprises a series of activities designed to develop self-awareness, the management of feelings, motivation, empathy and social skills and has had demonstrable positive effects promoting wellbeing and academic achievement (Hallam, 2009). Some children might also receive one-to-one play support from specialists trained in the developmental and therapeutic potential of play to promote holistic development. Rather than being remedial (as in the case of play therapy), this type of support is often preventative, working towards expanding the child's play skills to increase resilience and emotional health and subsequently enhancing cognitive, language, social, and/or physical development.

Play therapy grew from the psychoanalytic tradition of Freud (1856–1939). Anna Freud developed her father's ideas, documenting the benefits of play to establish a relationship between the therapist and the child that could facilitate the process of psychotherapy. In addition, she suggested children used play to replay events and explore ways of dealing with emotions. Melanie Klein placed even greater emphasis on the interpretation of children's play as being indicative of conflict or crises. A major criticism of psychoanalytic play therapy is the notion that play is representative of the unconscious mind and requires interpretation. There are real dangers associated with mis/over-interpretation or, indeed, whether any level of interpretation is warranted. Winnicott (1971) suggested that the process of play was far more important. This, coupled with the emergence of more humanistic approaches to therapy, has led to a variety of play therapy practices that are distinct from the psychoanalytic tradition, each involving different degrees of adult direction and interpretation (see Wilson & Ryan, 2005).

Therapeutic play

The value placed by Sheridan on children's spontaneous play accords with the non-directive approach developed by Axline (1989). This emphasizes both the significance of the play process and the importance of a warm and accepting therapeutic relationship. This approach is guided by eight principles that ensure the child feels their own initiated play activities are valued. The therapist recognizes this by reflecting back to the child what is being done, showing they are present and aware. There is acknowledgement but not praise, which ensures that the play proceeds in the way the child wishes, rather than promoting any compliance to social desirability. Whereas therapies following the psychoanalytic tradition can be difficult to evidence, more support is available for the beneficial effects of this non-directive approach. The non-directive approach supports not only children's emotional needs but the development of play skills. After ten sessions of non-directive play therapy, Trostle (1988) observed not only improvements in children's emotional health but more complex imaginative play. According to Jennings' EPR model (1999), this shift in play pattern would suggest increased self-awareness and the understanding of others.

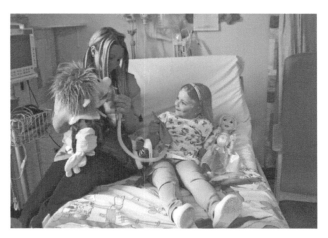 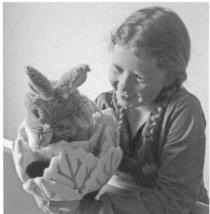

Puppets are a valuable resource for play professionals across educational, recreational and therapeutic contexts.

In play therapy, play is the language by which children communicate, explore and resolve issues that may be impacting on their lives. These issues might include developmental or organic problems, adjustment problems or moderate psycho-social crises. Some play therapists are also trained in psychotherapy, which allows them to consider children with more complex life histories or clinical issues. Observation and assessment skills are crucial for both the therapy process and appropriate referral. In contrast to other play professions, the focus of the work is the child's inner world, accessed in one-to-one therapy sessions, and the therapist avoids seeing the child in any other context so as not to confuse the relationship (McMahon, 2009). The profession is relatively new but is represented by professional organizations across the world. Play therapy is often a second career and training is generally restricted to those who have previous experience in working with children in some other capacity.

Therapeutic play professionals – Play therapists and therapeutic play specialists

Mary, play therapist, UK

I have been a play therapist for eight years but have worked with children for considerably longer, having originally trained as a social worker. My days are varied, involving meetings with other professionals, assessments and work for the courts in addition to direct work with the children. In the play sessions we might use puppets, clay, sand and water. I might end up being a noisy dinosaur or a crying baby when the children involve me in their role play. The best part of my job is knowing that the children trust me to help them through bad times. I reassure them they are safe and help them to feel empowered about their future. The job is challenging on lots of levels. I often have to convince other adults about the value of play as a way for children to communicate how they are feeling.

There are parallels between non-directive play therapy and good practice in other professional contexts. Emphasis is placed on the play process (maintaining the child's own cycle of play by responding to cues as described in chapter 1) and the naturally occurring therapeutic effects children's own spontaneous play activity can offer. Arguably, any setting where children are allowed to play freely, following their own intention, will offer the therapeutic effects encompassed in Axline's approach. This underpins the proposition of Hyder (2005), who argues that, for many children, the challenge of adversity can often be met with opportunities to play rather than therapy. Specialist knowledge about the process of play and its developmental and therapeutic potential can be utilized across a range of contexts to enhance children's development and address delays, imbalance, organic difficulties or the consequences of early play deprivation. As we have seen earlier, this might occur in schools or, as in the case below, through play sessions provided for children who have been exposed to domestic violence.

Trish, developmental and therapeutic play specialist, UK

I work as a developmental and therapeutic play specialist for Women's Aid. On a typical day, I could have two or three outreach appointments to visit children or young people in school for therapeutic play support. I take a mobile play kit, and the children choose what they'd like to do. The sessions are always child-led, and it works really well. This may be the only aspect of their chaotic lives where the child or young person has control. In the afternoon, I run creative play sessions for small groups of children within the refuge. It's great to watch the children's self-esteem grow, to see them overcome some of the challenges they've faced and enjoy themselves in play. Funding is very poor, though. I am the only children's and young people's worker within the organization, and I am pushed for time. I receive referrals on a daily basis.

A further context where therapeutic play is likely to occur is within a hospital setting. The first hospital play staff were employed in 1957 by St Bartholomew's and St Thomas' hospitals in London. Over the next two decades, the amount of staff employed in hospitals to support children's play grew significantly and, in 1972, the National Association of Hospital Play was established. While the initial focus was on providing opportunities for play while children were hospitalized, the role has grown considerably in scope and complexity over time. Hospital play specialists support children's holistic development during times of sickness and hospitalization, but also utilize focused interventions to prepare children for hospital procedures (Morgan & Howard, 2014). Their observations of children's play are also used to support clinical judgements.

Ann, hospital play specialist, UK

I trained as a hospital play specialist ten years ago, having worked for twelve years as a nursery nurse on the special care baby unit. I have been in my current post on the pediatric ward for eight years. I am one of three hospital play specialists who, with five play-leaders, make up our play team. We work closely with the nursing and medical staff and other members of the multidisciplinary team. Play has a special function in the hospital environment. It reduces anxiety, aids in assessment and diagnosis as well as speeding up recovery and rehabilitation. The children are not only ill but are separated from their friends and familiar surroundings. Play can really make a difference, helping children to understand and cope with treatment and illness. As well as organizing daily play activities in the playroom or at the bedside, we use play as a therapeutic tool, as in the preparation of children for theatre and other hospital procedures. I am based on the busy medical ward with ages ranging from birth to sixteen. No day is ever the same. I might start the day spending time with a toddler with food aversions – we use different tactile stimulation in the form of food or messy play. Another part of the day may be taken up with working with a child who is needle-phobic, preparing him for the necessary cannulation prior to his tonsil operation. Or I may be talking to a teenager who thinks life is not worth living after a row with her boyfriend. No one can say this job is boring or run of the mill.

Cohen (2006) suggests that the provision of recreational play spaces such as parks and playgrounds grew out of initiatives designed for social engineering. He describes how playgrounds were initially provided to keep children off the streets, offering places where they could engage in purposeful physical and social activity. The emphasis was on needing to control children's urge to play so as to avoid moral decline. In the 1930s, however, rather than being driven by any psychological, pedagogical or social outcome, Sorenson, a Danish landscaper, questioned whether society could do more to facilitate children's play needs and designed the first junk playground. It housed waste materials such as timber, old cars and boxes.

Recreational play

The first adventure playground was opened in 1943 in Denmark. Following its success, there was a prolific growth in playground provision. The opportunistic visit of Lady Allen of Hurtwood to the Danish junk playground in 1946 led to the adoption of the idea in the United Kingdom. These playgrounds came to be known as

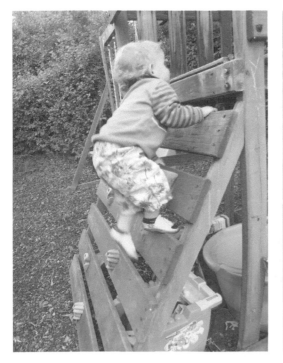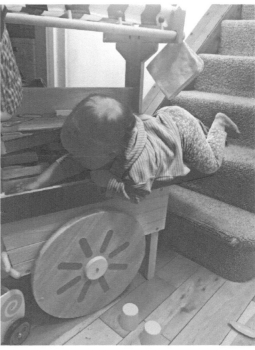

Not long after they are able to walk, these two young infants enjoy the risk of climbing.

adventure playgrounds and were characterized by affording children the opportunity to play as freely as possible within safe limits. The adventure playground movement recognized the need for children to satisfy their spontaneous drive to play and understood that play was necessarily child directed. Children needed outdoor spaces to take risks and try out new ideas, free from unnecessary rules and constraint. Children's ownership of the play was of principal importance, and this underpins current playwork practice.

On the trampoline, after spending time bouncing as high as they could, note how the overhanging branch afforded the girls an even more difficult challenge.

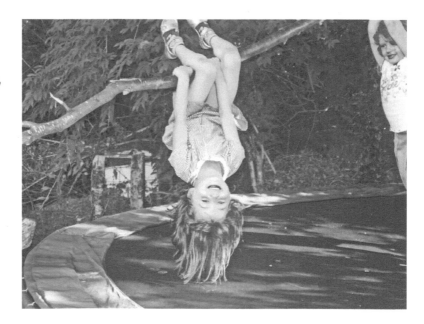

Gill (2007) suggests that opportunities for outdoor play might have become reduced in modern Western society due to increased traffic, media scare stories about pedophilia and ever-increasing concerns about litigation among professionals who work with children. Gray (2011) attributes a decline in children's opportunities for free play to a plethora of developmental and health concerns including, for example, decreased physical activity and weight concerns, depression and anxiety. Despite increasing evidence for the benefits of recreational play opportunities (Gill, 2014), and that play features as an important element of provision in policy documentation relating to children's services across domains (e.g. APPG, 2015; WAG,

2015), financial support to ensure sustainable, quality recreational play services for children appears in decline.

The play activity that frequently occurs in outdoor spaces contributes greatly to bodily awareness, balance and co-ordination (Greenland, 2006). Tovey (2010) describes how flexible play spaces promote risk-taking behaviour and allow children to explore the unknown. She proposes that managing risk is an essential, transferable life skill. A principal benefit of outdoor play is arguably the fact that it has reduced or self-regulated boundaries, which maximize children's sense of freedom, choice and control.

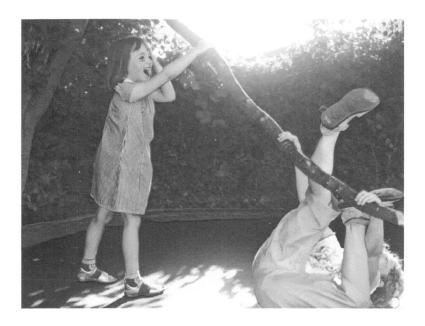

Playwork is rooted in the belief that children's opportunity to play has been curtailed by modern society. Playworkers are guided by a set of principles that emphasize the freedom and spontaneity of play and as such there is a focus on open-access provision, where children can come and go as they please. Playworkers use their extensive knowledge of play to provide and enrich spaces where children can engage in activities within safe boundaries. Emphasizing children's ownership of the play, their role is often facilitative and is never directed towards a particular outcome. Positions might include

Recreational play professionals – Playworkers and play development officers

work within out-of-school clubs, holiday play schemes or adventure playgrounds. Teams of playworkers might be co-ordinated by a play development officer, usually an experienced playworker who has undergone additional training.

Jo, play development officer, UK

I've been a play development officer with the local authority for five and a half years. I started with a playwork certificate but have since completed a variety of additional qualifications in community development, Forest School and youth work. I also have a master's degree in play, which extends my skills. Every day as a development officer throws up a new challenge. Variety keeps the job fresh, and although I have an office base, I work at different locations to deliver training, attend meetings, run events and act as an advocate for play. All this in addition to co-ordinating the open-access play schemes and my teams of playworkers. I meet lots of different people and like to see the positive contribution that our work has on communities. People often don't recognize the importance of play, particularly risky play, for children's healthy and happy development. With the current climate of fear towards strangers, increased traffic and a perceived lack of tolerance for playing children in the community, it's particularly difficult to win people over in terms of how vital it is. You really have to believe in what you do and have a thorough knowledge of the benefits for both the children and their communities. It's not easy to change people's beliefs, and sometimes it's frustrating.

Summary

- The best materials for play are often those that are the simplest.

- Space and time for play should not be unnecessarily constrained.

- Early relationships are particularly important for the development of secure attachments and the development of the growing brain.

- Children's friendships develop through play as they begin to appreciate characteristics about themselves and others.

- Adults can take a variety of roles in children's play but it is important to maintain children's sense of control over the direction of the activity.

- Children's development can be supported through play by a variety of professionals who are unified in their understanding that the benefits of play are associated with enabling children a sense of autonomy, control and independence.

- What challenges might adults face when interacting in play?

- What kinds of boundaries do we impose on play? Are these always necessary?

- In what ways might we increase children's sense of choice and control in play?

 Give yourself some time to think

Broadhead, P. *et al.* (2010). *Play and learning in the early years: From research to practice*. London: SAGE.

David, T. G., & Weinstein, C. S. (eds.). (2013). *Spaces for children: The built environment and child development*. London: Springer Science & Business Media.

Kilvington, J., & Wood, A. (2009). *Reflective playwork: For all who work with children*. London: Continuum.

Moyles, J. (2014). *The excellence of play, 4th ed.* Maidenhead: Open University Press.

Prendiville, E., & Howard, J. (2015). *Play therapy today*. London: Routledge.

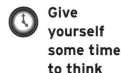 **Useful reading**

Useful play links

4Children

A national organization promoting play and out-of-school care facilities for all children: www.4children.org.uk

Action for Leisure

Information about accessible and appropriate play and leisure for disabled people of all ages: www.actionforleisure.org.uk

British Association of Play Therapy

Offers training routes in play therapy: www.bapt.info

Community Playthings

A useful website with lots of information on the benefits of different play activities: www.communityplaythings.co.uk

Fair Play for Children

Informative site that promotes children's right to play: www.fairplayforchildren.org

International Play Association

An international non-governmental organization that aims to protect, preserve and promote the child's right to play: http://ipaworld.org

Irish Association of Play Therapy and Psychotherapy

A professional association for play therapy, therapeutic play and psychotherapy: www.iapt.net

Kids Active

Advice and information relating to play for children with disabilities and special needs: www.kidsactive.org.uk

National Association of Hospital Play Staff

The professional organization for hospital play specialists: www.nahps.org.uk

National Children's Bureau

An organization dedicated to ensuring children's wellbeing: www.ncb.org.uk

Play Board

Supporting and resourcing play provision in Northern Ireland: www.playboard.org

Play England

An organization supporting children's play in England: www.playengland.org.uk

Play Scotland

An organization supporting children's play in Scotland: www.playscotland.org

Play Wales

An organization supporting children's play in Wales: www.playwales.org.uk

Playing Out

An organization that provides advice and support to communities to facilitate street play: http://playingout.net

PTUK

Offers training routes in play therapy: www.playtherapy.org.uk

Right to Play

Supports play provision for children internationally: www.rightto
play.org.uk

The Association for the Study of Play

A multidisciplinary organization whose purpose is to promote the
study of play: www.tasplay.org

References

All-Party Parliamentary Group (APPG) (2015). *Play — A Report by the All-Party Parliamentary Group on a Fit and Healthy Childhood*. London: APPG.

Axline, V. (1989). *Play Therapy*. Edinburgh: Churchill Livingstone.

Baillargeon, R. & DeVos, J. (1991). 'Object permanence in young infants: Further evidence'. *Child Development*, 1227–46.

Bateman, A., Danby, S. & Howard, J. (2013). 'Living in a broken world: How young children's wellbeing is supported through playing out their earthquake experiences'. *International Journal of Play*, 2(3), 202–19, doi:10.1080/21594937.2013.860270.

Boekee, K. & Brown, T. (2015). 'Gender stereotypes of children's toys: Investigating the perspectives of adults who have and do not have children'. *Journal of Occupational Therapy, Schools, & Early Intervention*, 8(1), 97–107.

Brockman, R., Jago, R. & Fox, K. (2011). 'Children's active play; Self-reported motivators, barriers and facilitators'. BMC Public Health, 11: 461.

Brown, F (2003). 'Compound flexibility, the role of playwork in child development'. In Brown, F. (ed.) *Playwork: Theory and Practice*. Buckingham: Open University Press.

Bruner, J. S. (1960). *The Process of Education*. New York: Vintage Books.

Bruner, J. S. (1979). *On Knowing: Essays for the Left Hand*. Cambridge, MA: Harvard University Press.

Brussoni, M., Olsen, L. L., Pike, I. & Sleet, D. A. (2012). 'Risky play and children's safety: Balancing priorities for optimal child development'. *International Journal of Environmental Research and Public Health*, 9(9), 3134–48.

Bryce, D. & Whitebread, D. (2012). 'The development of metacognitive skills: Evidence from observational analysis of young children's behaviour during problem-solving'. *Metacognition and Learning*, 7: 197–217.

Bundy, A. C. (1993). 'Assessment of play and leisure: delineation of the problem'. *American Journal of Occupational Therapy*, 47(3), 217–22.

Canning, N. (2013). 'Where's the bear? Over there! — Creative thinking and imagination in den making'. *Early Child Development and Care*, 183(8), 1042–53.

Chappell, K., Craft, A., Burnard, P. & Cremin, T. (2008). 'Question-posing and question responding: The heart of possibility thinking in the early years'. *Early Years: An International Journal of Research and Development*, 28(3), 267–286.

Children Schools and Families Committee (CSFC) (2010). The Training of Teachers – Fourth Report of Session 2009–10, Vol. 1. House of Commons, London: CSFC.

Cohen, D. (2006). *The Development of Play* (3rd ed.). Oxford: Routledge.

Cooney, M. & Sha, J. (1999). 'Play in the day of Qiaoqiao: A Chinese perspective'. *Child Study Journal*, 29, 97–111.

Cox, M. V. (2013). Children's Drawings of the Human Figure. Psychology Press.

Craft, A. (2005). *Creativity in Schools: Tensions and Dilemmas*. Oxford: Routledge.

Csikszentmihalyi, I. & Csikszentmihalyi M. (1988). *Optimal Experience: Psychological Studies of Flow in Consciousness*. New York: Cambridge University Press.

David, T. & Powell, S. (2005). 'Play in the early years: The influence of cultural difference'. In J. Moyles (ed.) *The Excellence of Play* (2nd ed.). Maidenhead: Open University Press.

Department for Children, Education, Lifelong Learning and Skills (DCELLS) (2008). *Foundation Phase in Wales*. Cardiff: Welsh Assembly Government.

Department for Culture, Media and Sport (2000). *Best Play*. London: National Playing Fields Association.

Department for Education and Skills (DfES) (2001). *Special Educational Needs Code of Practice*. Nottingham: HMSO.

Dowling, M. (2000). *Young Children's Personal, Social and Emotional Development*. London: SAGE.

Eisele, G. & Howard, J. (2012). 'Exploring the presence of characteristics associated with play within the ritual repetitive behaviour of autistic children'. *International Journal of Play*, 1(2), 139 doi:10.1080/21594 937.2012.692202.

Engelen, L., Bundy, A. C., Naughton, G., Simpson, J. M., Bauman, A., Ragen, J., . . . & Schiller, W. (2013). 'Increasing physical activity in young primary school children — it's child's play: A cluster randomised controlled trial'. *Preventive Medicine*, 56(5), 319–25.

Epstein, A. S., Schweinhart, L. J., DeBruin-Parecki, A., & Robin, K. B. (2004). 'Preschool assessment: A guide to developing a balanced approach.' *Preschool Policy Matters* 7, 1–2.

Erikson, E. (1963). *Childhood and Society*. New York: Norton.

Fearn, M. & Howard, J. (2011). 'Play as a resource for children facing adversity: An exploration of indicative case studies'. *Children and Society*, doi: 10.1111/j.1099-0860.2011.00357.

Gascoyne, S. (2012). Treasure Baskets and Beyond: Realizing the Potential of Sensory-Rich Play. McGraw-Hill Education.

Gill, T. (2007). *No Fear: Growing Up in a Risk Averse Society*. London: Calouste Gulbenkian Foundation.

Gill, T. (2014) 'The play return: A review of the wider impacts of play initiatives'. Children's Play Policy Forum.

Goldschmied, E. & Jackson, S. (1994) *People under Three: Young Children in Daycare*. London: Routledge.

Gosso, Y. (2010). 'Play in different cultures'. In P. Smith (ed.) *Children at Play* (80–98). West Sussex: Wiley Blackwell.

Goswami, U. (2014). *Cognition in Children*. Psychology Press.

Gray, P. (2011). 'The decline of play and the rise of psychopathology in children and adolescents'. *American Journal of Play*, 3(4), 443–63.

Greenland, P. (2006). 'Physical development'. In Bruce, T. (ed.) *Early Childhood: A Guide for Students*. London: SAGE.

Groos, K. (1901). *The Play of Man*. London: Heinemann.

Haight, W. L., Wang, X., Fung, H., Williams, H. & Mintz, J. (1999). 'Universal, developmental, and variable aspects of young children's play: A cross-cultural comparison of pretending at home'. *Child Development*, 70(6), 1477–88.

Halim, M. L., Ruble, D., Tamis-LeMonda, C. & Shrout, P. E. (2013). 'Rigidity in gender-typed behaviors in early childhood: A longitudinal study of ethnic minority children'. *Child Development*, 84(4), 1269–84.

Hall, G. S. (1920). *Youth*. New York: A. Appleton.

Hallam, S. (2009). 'An evaluation of the Social and Emotional Aspects of Learning (SEAL) programme: Promoting positive behaviour, effective learning and wellbeing in primary school children'. *Oxford Review of Education*, 35(3), 313–30.

Hamilton, G. (2016). Honouring Dr. Mary D. Sheridan. The Royal Society of Medicine Wall of Honour. Available online at www.rsm-wallofhonour.com (accessed 29 June 2016).

Holland, P. (2003). *We Don't Play with Guns Here: War, Weapon and Superhero Play in the Early Years*. Buckingham: Open University Press.

Holt, N. L., Lee, H., Millar, C. A. & Spence, J. C. (2015). 'Eyes on where children play: A retrospective study of active free play'. Children's Geographies, 13: 73–88.

Howard, J. (2002). 'Eliciting children's perceptions of play using the activity apperception story procedure'. *Early Child Development and Care*, 172(5), 489–502.

Howard, J. (2009). 'Play, learning and development in the early years'. In T. Maynard & N. Thomas (eds.) *An Introduction to Early Childhood Studies*. London: SAGE.

Howard, J. (2010a). 'The developmental and therapeutic value of children's play: Re-establishing teachers as play professionals'. In J. Moyles (ed.) *The Excellence of Play* (3rd ed.). Maidenhead: Open University Press.

Howard, J. (2010b). 'Making the most of play in the early years: Understanding and building on children's perceptions'. In P. Broadhead, J. Howard & E. Wood (eds.) *Play and Learning in Early Childhood: Research into Practice*. London: SAGE.

Howard, J. & McInnes, K. (2013a). *The Essence of Play: A Practice Companion for Professionals Working with Children and Young People*. Routledge.

Howard, J. & McInnes, K. (2013b). 'The impact of children's perception of an activity as play rather than not play on emotional well-being'. *Child: Care, Health and Development*, 39(5): 737–42, doi: 10.1111/j.1365-2214.2012.01405.x (Epub 6 June, 2012).

Howard. J. & Miles, G. (2008). 'Incorporating empirical findings that link play and learning into a behavioural threshold and fluency theory of play'. Paper presented at the BPS Psychology of Education Section Conference, Milton Keynes, November.

Howard-Jones, P. (2011). *The Impact of Digital Technologies on Human Wellbeing: Evidence from the Sciences of Mind and Brain*. Oxford.

Howard, J., Miles, G.E., Rees-Davies, L. and Bertenshaw, E.J. (2017) Play in Middle Childhood: Everyday Play Behaviour and Associated Emotions. *Children and Society*. ISSN 0951-0605, Online: 1099-0860 (In Press).

Hua, J., Duan, T., Gu, G., Wo, D., Zhu, Q., Liu, J. Q., . . . & Meng, W. (2016). 'Effects of home and education environments on children's motor performance in China'. *Developmental Medicine & Child Neurology*.

Hughes, B. (1999). *A Playworker's Taxonomy of Play Types*. London: PLAYLINK.

Hughes, F. (2010). *Children, Play and Development* (4th ed.). London: SAGE.

Hutt, C. (1976). 'Exploration and play in children'. In J. S. Bruner, A. Jolly & K. Sylva (eds.) *Play—Its Role in Development and Evolution*. New York: Basic Books.

Hyder, T. (2005). *War, Conflict and Play*. Maidenhead: Open University Press.

Hyun, E. (1998). *Making Sense of Developmentally and Culturally Appropriate Practice (DCAP) in Early Childhood Education*. New York: Peter Lang.

Isaacs, S. (1932). *The Social Development of Young Children: A Study of Beginnings*. London: Routledge and Kegan Paul.

Jarvis, P. (2006). 'Rough and tumble play: Lessons in life'. *Evolutionary Psychology*, 4, 330–46.

Jarvis, P., Newman, S. & Swiniarski, L. (2014). 'On "becoming social":

The importance of collaborative free play in childhood'. *International Journal of Play*, 3: 53–68.

Jennings, S. (1999). *An Introduction to Developmental Play Therapy.* London: Jessica Kingsley Press.

Jennings, S. (2011). Healthy Attachments and Neuro-Dramatic Play. London: Jessica Kingsley Press.

John, A., Halliburton, A. & Humphrey, J. (2013). 'Child-mother and child-father play interaction patterns with preschoolers'. *Early Child Development and Care*, 183(3–4), 483–97.

Kalliala, M. (2006). *Play Culture in a Changing World.* Maidenhead: Open University Press.

Kamp, K. (2015). 'Making children legitimate'. *The Archaeology of Childhood: Interdisciplinary Perspectives on an Archaeological Enigma*, SUNY Press.

Keating, I., Fabian, H., Jordan, P., Mavers, D. & Roberts, J. (2000). '"Well, I've not done any work today. I don't know why I came to school": perceptions of play in the reception class'. *Educational Studies*, 26(4), 437–54.

King, P. & Howard, J. (2014). 'Children's perceptions of choice in relation to their play at home, in the school playground and at the out-of-school club'. *Children and Society*, 28(2), 116–27, doi:10.1111/j.1099-0860.2012.00455.x.

Krasnor, L. R. & Pepler, D. J. (1980). 'The study of children's play: Some suggested future directions'. In K. H. Rubin (ed.) *New Directions for Child Development: Children's Play* (vol. 9). San Francisco: Jossey- Bass.

Laevers, F. (1994). *The Leuvens Involvement Scale for Young Children (LIC-YC).* Leuven, Belgium: Centre for Experiential Education.

Lester, S. & Russell, W. (2008). *Play for a Change. Play Policy and Practice: A Review of Contemporary Perspectives.* London: NCB and Play England.

Lester, S. & Russell, W. (2010). *Children's Right to Play: An Examination of the Importance of Play in the Lives of Children Worldwide.* The Hague: Bernard van Leer Foundation.

Li, Y., Coplan, R. J., Wang, Y., Yin, J., Zhu, J., Gao, Z. & Li, L. (2016). 'Preliminary evaluation of a social skills training and facilitated play early intervention programme for extremely shy young children in China'. *Infant and Child Development.*

Lieberman, J. N. (1977). *Playfulness: Its Relationship to Imagination and Creativity.* London: Academic Press.

Lillard, A. S., Lerner, M. D., Hopkins, E. J., Dore, R. A., Smith, E. D. & Palmquist, C. M. (2013). 'The impact of pretend play on children's development: A review of the evidence'. *Psychological Bulletin*, 139(1), 1.

Lindahl, L. B. & Heimann, M. (1997). Social proximity in early mother infant interactions: implications for gender differences? *Early Development and Parenting*, 6(2), 83–88.

Lindon, J. (2001). *Understanding Children's Play*. Cheltenham: Nelson Thornes.

Lindsey, E. W., Cremeens, P. R. & Caldera, Y. M. (2010). 'Gender differences in mother-toddler and father-toddler verbal initiations and responses during caregiving and play context'. *Sex Roles*, 65(5–6), 399–411.

Lorch, M., & Hellal, P. (2010). Darwin's 'Natural Science of Babies'. *Journal of the History of the Neurosciences*, 19(2), 140–57.

Marschark, M. (1993). *Psychological Development of Deaf Children*. New York: Oxford University Press.

Maybin, J. & Woodhead, M. (2003). *Childhoods in Context*. Milton Keynes: Open University Press.

McInnes, K., Howard, J., Miles, G. & Crowley, K. (2009). 'Behavioural differences exhibited by children when practicing a task under formal and playful conditions'. *Educational and Child Psychology*, 26(2), 31–39.

McInnes, K., Howard, J., Miles, G. & Crowley, K. (2011). 'Differences in practitioners' understanding of play and how this influences pedagogy and children's perceptions of play'. Early Years 31 (2) 121–33.

McInnes, K., Howard, J., Miles, G. & Crowley, K. (2013). 'The nature of adult-child interaction in the early years classroom: Implications for children's perceptions of play and subsequent learning behaviour'. *European Early Childhood Education Research Journal*, 21(2), 268–82.

McMahon, L. (2009). *The Handbook of Play Therapy and Therapeutic Play* (2nd ed.). Sussex: Routledge.

Meltzoff, A. N. & Moore, M. K. (1997). 'Explaining facial imitation: A theoretical model'. *Early Development and Parenting*, 6, 179–92.

Meltzoff, A. N., Williamson, R. A. & Marshall, P. J. (2013). 'Developmental perspectives on action science: Lessons from infant imitation and cognitive neuroscience'. In W. Prinz, M. Beisert & A. Herwig (eds.), *Action Science: Foundations of an Emerging Discipline* (281–306). Cambridge: MIT Press.

Michel, G. F., Campbell, J. M., Marcinowski, E. C., Nelson, E. L. & Babik, I. (2016). 'Infant hand and the development of cognitive abilities'. *Frontiers in Psychology*, 7.

Miller, E. & Kuhaneck, H. (2008). 'Children's perceptions of play experiences and the development of play preferences: A qualitative study'. American Journal of Occupational Therapy, 62: 407–15.

Milteer, R. M., Ginsburg, K. R., Mulligan, D. A., Ameenuddin, N., Brown, A., Christakis, D. A., . . . & Levine, A. E. (2012). 'The importance of play in promoting healthy child development and maintaining strong parent-child bond: Focus on children in poverty'. *Pediatrics*, 129 (1), e204–13.

Moyles, J. (1989). *Just Playing?: Role and Status of Play in Early Childhood Education*. Buckingham: Open University Press.

Nicholson, S. (1971). 'The theory of loose parts'. *Landscape Architecture Quarterly*, 62(1), 30–34.

O'Reilly, A. W. & Bornstein, M. H. (1993). 'Caregiver-child interaction in play'. In M. H. Bornstein & A. W. O'Reilly (eds.) *The Role of Play in the Development of Thought*. San Francisco: Jossey-Bass.

Parker, C. J. (2007). *Children's Perceptions of a Playful Environment: Contextual, Social and Environmental Differences*. Unpublished thesis, University of Glamorgan.

Parten, M. B. (1932). 'Social participation among preschool children'. *Journal of Abnormal and Social Psychology*, 27, 243–69.

Patrick, G. T. (1916). *The Psychology of Relaxation*. Boston: Houghton-Mifflin.

Pellegrini, A. (1991). *Applied Child Study: A Developmental Approach*. New Jersey: Lawrence Erlbaum.

Pellegrini, A. D. & Gustafson, K. (2005). Boys' and girls' uses of objects for exploration, play and tools in early childhood. In A. D. Pellegrini, & P. K. Smith (eds.).*The Nature of Play: Great Apes and Humans* (113–35). New York: Guilford Press.

Perry, B., Hogan, L. & Marlin, S. (2000). 'Curiosity, pleasure, and play: A neurodevelopmental perspective'. *Haaeyc Advocate*. 20: 9–12.

Piaget, J. (1951). *Play, Dreams and Imitation in Childhood*. London: Routledge and Kegan Paul.

Plowman, L. & McPake, J. (2013). 'Seven myths about young children and technology'. *Childhood Education*, 89(1), 27–33.

Ring, K. (2010). 'Supporting a playful approach to drawing'. In P. Broadhead, J. Howard & E. Wood (eds.) *Play and Learning in the Early Years*. London: SAGE.

Robson, S. (1993). '"Best of all I like choosing time": Talking with children about play and work'. *Early Child Development and Care*, 92, 37–51.

Rogoff, B. (2003). *The Cultural Nature of Human Development*. New York: Oxford University Press.

Roopnarine, J. L. (2012). 'What is the state of play?' *International Journal of Play*, 1(3), 228–30.

Roopnarine, J. L., Lasker, J., Sacks, M. & Stores, M. (1998). 'The cultural contents of children's play'. In O. N. Saracho & B. Spodek (eds.) *Multiple Perspectives on Play in Early Childhood Education*. New York: State University of New York Press.

Saracho, O. N. (1990). *Cognitive Style and Early Education*. New York: Gordon & Breach: Science Publishers.

Servin, A., Bohlin, G. & Berlin, L. (1999). 'Sex differences in 1-, 3-, and 5-year-olds' toy-choice in a structured play-session'. *Scandinavian Journal of Psychology*, 40, 43–48.

Sheridan, M. (1977). *Spontaneous Play in Early Childhood: From Birth to Six Years* (1st ed.). Windsor: NFER.

Sobel, D. (2001). *Children's Special Places: Exploring the Role of Forts, Dens and Bush Houses in Middle Childhood*. Detroit: Wayne State University Press.

Spencer, H. (1898). *Principles of Psychology*. New York: Appleton.

Sturrock, G. & Else, P. (1998). 'The playground as therapeutic space: Playwork as healing [known as 'The Colorado Paper']'. In G. Sturrock & P. Else (2005) *Therapeutic Playwork Reader One*. Sheffield: Ludemos.

Sutton-Smith, B. (1974). *How to Play with Your Children (and When Not to)*. New York: Hawthorne Press.

Sylva, K., Melhuish, E., Sammons, P., Siraj-Blatchford, I. & Taggart, B. (eds.). (2010). *Early Childhood Matters: Evidence from the Effective Pre-school and Primary Education Project*. Routledge.

Tovey, H. (2007). *Playing Outdoors: Spaces and Places, Risks and Challenge (Debating Play)*. Maidenhead: Open University Press.

Tovey, H. (2010). 'Playing on the edge: Perceptions of risk and danger in outdoor play'. In P. Broadhead, J. Howard & E. Wood (eds.), *Play and Learning in the Early Years*. London: SAGE.

Trostle, S. L. (1988). 'The effects of child-centred group play sessions on social-emotional growth of three- to six-year-old bilingual Puerto Rican children'. *Journal of Research in Childhood Education*, 3(2), 93–106.

United Nations (1989). *Convention on the Rights of the Child*. Brussels: United Nations Assembly.

Vygotsky, L. S. (1978). *Mind in Society, the Development of Higher Mental Psychological Processes*. Cambridge: Harvard University Press.

Watson-Gegeo, K. A. (2001). 'Fantasy and reality: The dialectic of work and play in Kwara'ae children's lives'. *Ethos*, 29(2), 138–58.

Webb, N. B. (2013). Culturally Diverse Parent-Child and Family Relationships: A Guide for Social Workers and Other Practitioners. Columbia University Press.

Webb, S. & Brown, F. (2003). 'Playwork in adversity: Working with abandoned children in Romania'. In F. Brown (ed.) *Playwork Theory and Practice*. Buckingham: Open University Press.

Weisgram, E. S., Fulcher, M. & Dinella, L. M. (2014). 'Pink gives girls permission: Exploring the roles of explicit gender labels and gender-typed colors on preschool children's toy preferences'. *Journal of Applied Developmental Psychology*, 35(5), 401–9.

Welsh Assembly Government (WAG) (2015). Child Poverty Strategy for Wales. WAG.

Whitebread, D. (2010). 'Play, metacognition and self regulation'. In P. Broadhead, J. Howard & E. Wood (eds.), *Play and Learning in the Early Years*. London: SAGE.

Whitebread, D. (2012). *The Importance of Play: A Report on the Value of Children's Play with Policy Recommendations*. Brussels: Toys Industry Europe.

Wilson, R. (2012). *Nature and Young Children: Encouraging Creative Play and Learning in Natural Environments*. Routledge.

Wilson, K. & Ryan, V. (2005). *Play Therapy: A Non-directive Approach for Children and Adolescents* (2nd ed.). London: Elsevier Science.

Winnicott, D. W. (1971). *Playing and Reality*. London: Tavistock Publications.

Wooldridge, M. B. & Shapka, J. (2012). 'Playing with technology: Mother-toddler interaction scores lower during play with electronic toys'. *Journal of Applied Developmental Psychology*, 33(5), 211–18.

Yang, Y. (2013). 'A qualitative study of teachers' involvement in children's play'. *Literacy Information and Computer Education Journal*, 4(4), 1153–60.

Yavuz, L. C. 'The effects of loose parts and nature-based play on creativity in the Montessori early childhood (3–6-year-old) classroom' (2016). Masters of Arts in Education Action Research Papers. Paper 141.

Index

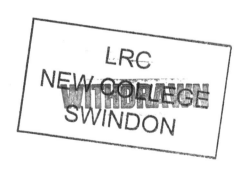